I0617477

THE ULTIMATE PREPPER PANTRY SURVIVAL GUIDE

90 DAYS OF NUTRITIONAL SURVIVAL FOOD TO STOCKPILE ENSURING YOUR FAMILY'S SAFETY DURING A CATASTROPHE

CARLOS MACK

THE ULTIMATE PREPPER PANTRY SURVIVAL GUIDE

90 DAYS OF NUTRITIONAL SURVIVAL FOOD TO
STOCKPILE ENSURING YOUR FAMILY'S SAFETY
DURING A CATASTROPHE

CARLOS MACK

CONTENTS

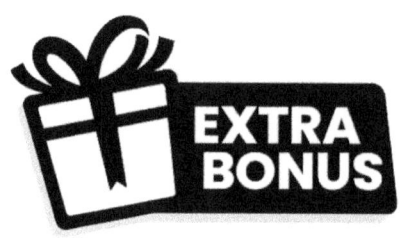

Thank you for embarking on this literary journey with me! Your support and enthusiasm for my book mean the world. As a token of gratitude, I'm thrilled to offer you exclusive access to the "Ultimate Prepper Pantry Inventory Calculator Spreadsheet." Simply scan the QR code below and drop your email to receive this invaluable tool – no strings attached, just a little something extra for being a loyal reader. Your continued support is truly appreciated, and I hope this bonus enriches your prepping journey in the most extraordinary ways!

SCAN THE QR CODE BELOW

SCAN ME

INTRODUCTION

A NEW DAWN OF PREPAREDNESS

In the darkest hours of unforeseen turmoil, when chaos reigns, and uncertainty looms, the weight of unpreparedness bears down upon the soul. It's the chilling realization that the tomorrow we once took for granted may never arrive, leaving us in a world defined by survival. The panic that ensues, the fear that grips our hearts, and the helplessness we feel in the face of the unknown can be paralyzing. It's a pain you know all too well—the fear for your family's safety, the anxiety over what tomorrow may bring, and the sense of vulnerability in a world that seems more unpredictable by the day.

But amidst this uncertainty, there is a path to resilience, a beacon of hope, and a strategy to overcome the crushing weight of unpreparedness. It's a future where you and your loved ones no longer need to live in fear but can embrace each day with the confidence that comes from being ready for anything. This is the promise of "The Ultimate Prepper Pantry Survival Guide: 90 Days of Nutritional Survival Food to Stockpile Ensuring Your Family's Safety During a Catastrophe". Written as a guide designed to transform fear into strength, vulnerability into preparedness, and chaos into control.

In the pages of this book, you will embark on a transformative journey. You will learn the art of building a prepper pantry that ensures your family's well-being in the face of any catastrophe. You will discover the power of proactive preparedness and the security that comes from having a stockpile of essential supplies. More importantly, you will be equipped with the knowledge and tools to paint a brighter, safer future for your loved ones.

But why should you listen to me? What makes me an authority on preparedness and survival? For years, I have delved into the world of prepping, drawing upon my extensive research and first-hand experience to compile the most comprehensive, practical, and actionable guides. My expertise is not rooted in fear mongering but in a genuine desire to empower families like yours to navigate crises with grace and strength. This marks my fifth book dedicated to prepping and survival. Each of the previous four attained the coveted #1 new release badge on Amazon. Am I an expert in survival and prepping? I staunchly believe that claiming expertise is a limitation; there's a perpetual wealth of knowledge to pursue. I do, however, profess an unwavering passion for prepping and an insatiable appetite for continual learning.

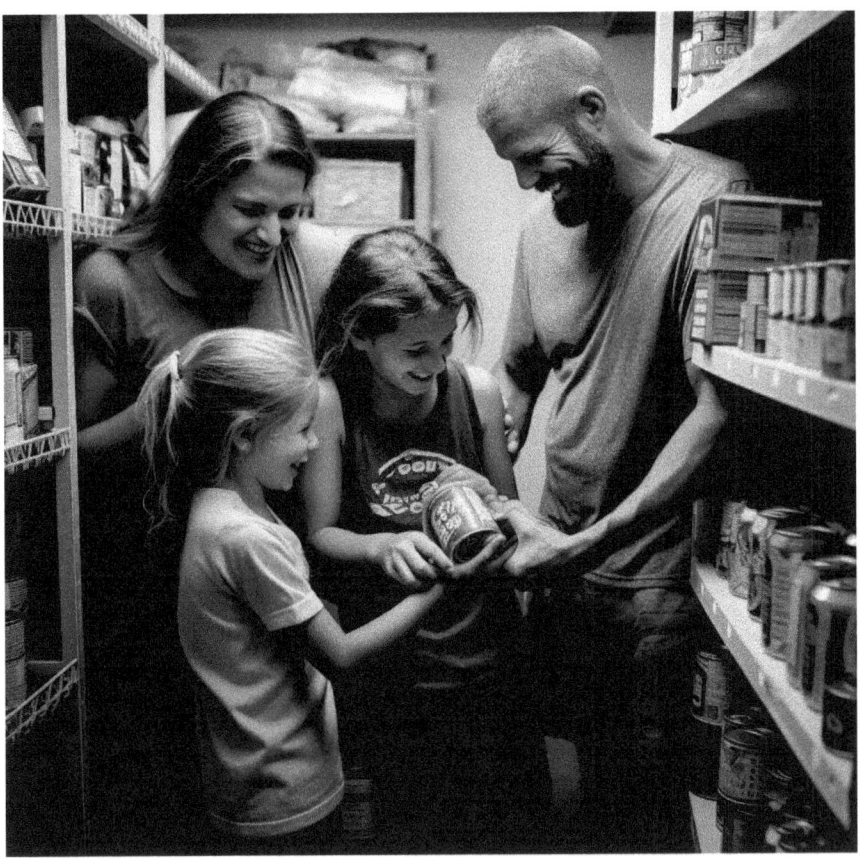

With a clear, empathetic understanding of the pain and anxiety that unpreparedness can bring, I am uniquely poised to guide you toward a better future. There's no better moment than now to confront this issue. Let today be the day when the insights and strategies that have empowered numerous families—turning fearful, unprepared individuals into proactive, resilient units—equip you to confront whatever challenges may arise ahead of you!

As you set forth on this path through "The Ultimate Prepper Pantry Survival Guide," you will discover the secrets of stockpiling nutritional survival food, ensuring your family's safety even in the direst of circumstances. From the fundamentals of creating a prepper pantry tailored to your family's unique needs to the nuances of maintaining nutritional balance and variety, this guide is your roadmap to preparedness and peace of mind.

So, embrace this opportunity to leave behind the pain of unpreparedness. Imagine a future where your family thrives, where your loved ones stand strong, and where your home becomes a fortress of security and comfort. This isn't a path meant to be traversed alone, instead, it's a path we'll navigate together, with me as your guide. The path to resilience starts here, and your destiny of preparedness is waiting to be realized within these pages.

THE PILLARS OF SURVIVAL FOOD STOCKPILING AND CATASTROPHE PREPAREDNESS: FROM CHAOS TO CONFIDENCE

"In times of crisis, the wise build bridges, while the foolish build barriers."

— T'CHALLA, BLACK PANTHER

A REAL-LIFE STORY

In the darkest days of Hurricane Katrina, a family found themselves trapped in their flooded home. With no access to food or clean water, they relied on the limited supplies they had stockpiled. These provisions, carefully stored away for emergencies, became a lifeline. The food stockpile sustained them through the crisis, allowing them to survive until help arrived. This real-life story highlights the significance of a well-planned food supply in times of catastrophe. It's a stark reminder that disaster can strike unexpectedly, and preparedness can make all the difference.

Core Principles of Food Stockpiling

Food stockpiling forms the bedrock of your catastrophe preparedness strategy. It's essential to understand the core principles that guide the process, ensuring that your stockpile is both practical and effective. The principles discussed in this chapter provide a solid framework for your journey into preparedness. The following core principles will be threaded throughout the book and examined in greater detail. As you accumulate knowledge, develop the right mindset, and assemble your provisions, you'll find yourself on the path to true self-reliance and peace of mind during any catastrophe.

LONG-TERM SUSTAINABILITY

The heart of food stockpiling is ensuring your family's sustenance during a catastrophe. This principle requires careful selection of non-perishable, long-lasting food items that can be stored for an extended period.

Examples of such items include:

- **Canned goods** - Cooked and sealed under high pressure with 2-5 years of shelf life, fruits, vegetables, meats, soups in cans are must-have items in your food stockpile.
- **Dried Grains** - I recommend keeping on hand a variety such as flax, barley, grits, quinoa, rye, millet etc (expert tip: don't overstock all of these grains if your family hates the taste of 1 or 2 of them, then they will just go to waste and take up valuable space.) Stored in airtight containers, these could last 10 years or more.
- **Legumes** - Dried, legumes can hang around for years and still taste great. Plus, they are one of the best sources of plant proteins around, packed with many vitamins and minerals. Here are some of our favorites: chickpeas, pinto beans, kidney beans, black beans, black-eyed peas, lentils (red, green, brown).
- **Flour** - Do you bake? Flour is an affordable and versatile ingredient you must stock up on.
- **Pasta** - Pasta is a foundational meal starter, with ridiculously long shelf-life. This is another of my family's favorites, plus it's so filling!
- **Dried Fruits** - Simple, delicious, nutritionally dense, and not a space hog. You're welcome!
- **Rice** - Would I be a "prepper expert" if I forgot rice? Most say it's #1 food on planet earth, plus it can net

you other products like: milk, flour, oil, alcohol, dessert, vinegar, cereal, even paper!

- **Nuts and Seeds** - These are nutritional heavy-weights for such small foods! Unless peanut allergies are present, keep several kinds in your stockpile. These are easy to grab for a BOB, or as a to-go snack when needed. Additional benefits; they are a longer lasting snack, and I see no harm in spitting the shells onto the ground when outside giving them back to nature. The birds and chipmunks will thank you.
- **Oats** - You can grind oats for flour, boil it for oatmeal, toast them, bake them into bread or muffins. There are so many useful ways to use oats, and like everything else on this list they have a nice shelf-life.
- **Honey** - Honey boasts an incredibly long shelf life due to its low water content and natural acidity, antibacterial properties. It's a fantastic snack eaten raw, added to drinks, used as a topping, or incorporated into cooking and baking for sweetness. Your pantry's sweet swiss army knife!
- **Peanut Butter** - One of my personal favorites, it boosts morale when a dull cracker or cold piece of bread receives this delicious companion!
- **Spices** - A day without sun is like food without spice - dull. More than the basics of salt, pepper, garlic powder, consider spices like ginger, cinnamon, and turmeric too. These spices not only are super

flavorful, they also possess magical health benefits to fight inflammation and improve your immune system. These will be discussed at length below.

- **Herbs** - Grown them yourself, then dry them, freeze them, all sorts of options that will give meals enhanced depth, and most importantly will be used for countless medicinal remedies for almost any ailment that your family would encounter.

I could have easily doubled this list, and had to stop for a quick snack from my own pantry while writing about these foods! Bottom line, a well-maintained stockpile can provide food for years, ensuring you're ready for various crises. It's important to note again, that different food items have varying shelf lives. For example, canned foods can last for several years, while dried grains and beans have a longer shelf life if stored correctly. Even the same food, preserved in different ways, has a different expiration. Think of an apple. A freshly picked apple lasts about 1-2 weeks. Dehydrated apples will last 6-12 months, maybe longer. Canned apples, preserved and stored correctly, can last over 2 years! Some say properly preserved, natural honey will never expire. I'll let you be the judge there. So regularly check the expiration dates and rotate items to use and replace, ensuring nothing goes to waste. We will discuss the 3-tier & FIFO methods for your pantry stock shortly. If you don't know what those are, I would suggest you keep reading.

FOOD GROUP REPRESENTATION FOR DIVERSIFIED NUTRITION

A well-rounded diet is essential for maintaining health during a crisis. Let's say you only have 100 lbs. of rice stored in your basement, with no other food stockpiled. That rice will sustain you, but it sure will get boring after several days! To cover all nutritional bases, your stockpile should include a variety of food groups, including proteins, carbohydrates, fats, and essential vitamins and minerals. A diverse range of foods ensures that your family receives a wide spectrum of essential nutrients, even in the absence of fresh produce. Here's a breakdown of these food groups, along with fresh and shelf-stable options for each:

Proteins

Proteins are crucial for various bodily functions, primarily known for their role in muscle maintenance and repair. During emergencies or crisis situations, maintaining muscle mass and overall body strength becomes vital for resilience. Sources such as canned meats, beans, and nut butter provide essential amino acids needed for these functions. A single adult's need for 50 to 60 grams of protein daily is critical for tissue repair, immune function, and hormone production.

During times of stress or injury, protein needs might increase to support healing and recovery. In emergencies, ensuring a consistent supply of proteins becomes essential, especially for those with health conditions like diabetes or metabolic disorders, where protein intake can influence blood sugar levels.

Fresh: Eggs, cheese, and canned or cured meats. These are excellent sources of protein and can be rotated for freshness.

Shelf-Stable: Canned beans, lentils, canned fish (such as tuna and salmon), and jerky. They provide protein, and many options are low in sodium for a healthier stockpile.

Carbohydrates

Carbohydrates serve as the primary energy source for the body. They're necessary for fueling daily activities and maintaining bodily functions. Stockpiling carbohydrates like rice and pasta ensures a readily available source of energy during challenging times. An adult's requirement of 225 to 325 grams of carbohydrates daily is essential for sustaining energy levels and supporting the central nervous system.

Individuals with conditions like diabetes need to manage their carbohydrate intake carefully to control blood sugar levels. During emergencies, balancing the need for energy from carbs while considering their impact on blood glucose becomes crucial.

Fresh: Sweet potatoes and corn. These offer carbohydrates, fiber, and essential vitamins and minerals.

Shelf-Stable: Shelf-stable bread, crackers, and cereals. Look for whole-grain options to maximize their nutritional value.

Fats and Oils

Fats and oils are vital components of a prepper's pantry for multiple reasons during emergencies. They serve as concentrated sources of energy, essential for maintaining body warmth and providing sustained fuel during physically demanding situations. In a food stockpile, they contribute to meal preparation, enhancing taste and texture while boosting the caloric density of stored foods. Shelf-stable oils like olive oil, coconut oil, or vegetable oils are crucial for cooking, preserving, and flavoring various dishes. Additionally, they aid in the absorption of fat-soluble vitamins, making them pivotal for ensuring the body can efficiently utilize the nutrients from the available food supply. Lastly, fats and oils can offer a sense of satiety and satisfaction, which is essential during times of rationing or limited food availability.

Fresh: Avocados and nuts like almonds and walnuts. These provide healthy fats and essential fatty acids.

Shelf-Stable: Olive oil, coconut oil, and shelf-stable nut butters. These fats remain stable over time and are essential for cooking and flavor.

Grains

Grains, the cornerstone of any well-prepared pantry, stand as critical components for numerous compelling reasons. Firstly, their long shelf life renders them superb for stockpiling, ensuring sustenance through prolonged periods of scarcity or emergencies. Their versatility in various forms—rice, wheat, oats, quinoa, and more—offers flexibility in meal preparation, catering to diverse dietary needs and culinary preferences. Rich in carbohydrates, grains serve as an energy powerhouse, providing the essential fuel needed for survival and maintaining optimal bodily functions, especially during high-stress situations. Furthermore, their nutritional density, encompassing crucial vitamins, minerals, and fiber, fortifies overall health and aids digestion, pivotal in maintaining resilience during unpredictable circumstances. Grains possess a role beyond mere sustenance; they contribute to a sense of normalcy, allowing for comforting, familiar meals even in the midst of turmoil, fostering stability and mental well-being. Hence, in the prepper's pantry, grains transcend mere sustenance; they symbolize resilience, adaptability, and the foundation of preparedness in times of adversity.

Fresh: Whole grains like brown rice, quinoa, whole wheat pasta, and barley. These provide complex carbohydrates, fiber, and various vitamins and minerals.

Shelf-Stable: Long-lasting options such as white rice, pasta, and various types of dried bread. Ensure that these are stored in airtight containers to prevent moisture and pests.

Fruits and Vegetables

Fruits and vegetables play a pivotal role in a prepper's pantry for several reasons in emergency food stockpiles. Firstly, they offer essential vitamins, minerals, and antioxidants critical for maintaining overall health and immunity, which can be compromised during stressful situations. Canned or freeze-dried fruits and vegetables provide long-term storage options without losing much of their nutritional value. Additionally, they introduce variety and flavor to an otherwise monotonous diet, boosting morale and mental well-being. Their fiber content aids in digestion and helps regulate blood sugar levels, which can be crucial during times of limited food availability or when relying on preserved or shelf-stable foods. Lastly, their versatility allows for different preparation methods, enhancing meal options and nutritional diversity in a survival scenario.

Fruits

Fresh: Apples, oranges, bananas, and hardy options like citrus fruits. Fresh fruits provide essential vitamins, minerals, and dietary fiber.

Shelf-Stable: Canned fruits (in water or natural juices) and dried fruits like raisins and apricots. These have a longer shelf life and retain their nutritional value.

Vegetables

Fresh: Root vegetables such as potatoes, carrots, and squash. These are not only nutritious but also have a relatively long shelf life in cool, dark storage.

Shelf-Stable: Canned vegetables (preferably low-sodium varieties) and dehydrated vegetable mixes. These retain their nutritional value and can be used in a variety of recipes.

Vitamins and Minerals: A variety of fruits and vegetables, even in dehydrated form, can provide essential vitamins and minerals. For example, vitamin C is vital for immune function, while calcium supports bone health. If not confined to pill bottles or suspended in tinctures, the vital nutrients of vitamins and minerals can spring to life in the bountiful gardens of your homestead. Further elaboration on this subject awaits in the subsequent sections for you green thumbs out there.

When calculating your stockpile, consider these nutritional needs for each family member to ensure that you are adequately providing for them. By offering a variety of foods that cover a broad spectrum of nutrients, you will help maintain physical health, boost immunity, and keep your family well-nourished during challenging times.

Balancing the intake of these macronutrients, considering individual health conditions, and ensuring a diverse supply of these essential nutrients in emergency stockpiles becomes fundamental for maintaining health, energy, and resilience during challenging times.

Vitamins and Minerals

Fresh: Many Vitamin A (carrots, sweet potatoes, spinach, kale), Vitamin C (oranges, strawberries, bell peppers), Vitamin K (broccoli), B Vitamins (meat, poultry, dairy, eggs, leafy greens), Vitamin E (nuts, seeds, vegetable oils)

Shelf stable: Vitamin D, Zinc, Vitamin C, Magnesium, Vitamin B12, Iron, Calcium just a few pill bottles we have in reserve.

SUPPLEMENTING YOUR STOCKPILE WITH VITAMINS AND MINERALS

To address potential nutrient gaps in your stockpile and ensure your family's optimal health, consider supplementing with vitamins and minerals. Here are long-lasting options suitable for stockpiling, along with recommended dosages:

Multivitamins: A general multivitamin can help cover essential nutrient needs during an emergency. Ensure you select long-lasting options with expiration dates well into the future.

Vitamin C: Vitamin C tablets or powder can be stored for their immune-boosting properties. A daily dose of 500-1,000 mg is generally recommended.

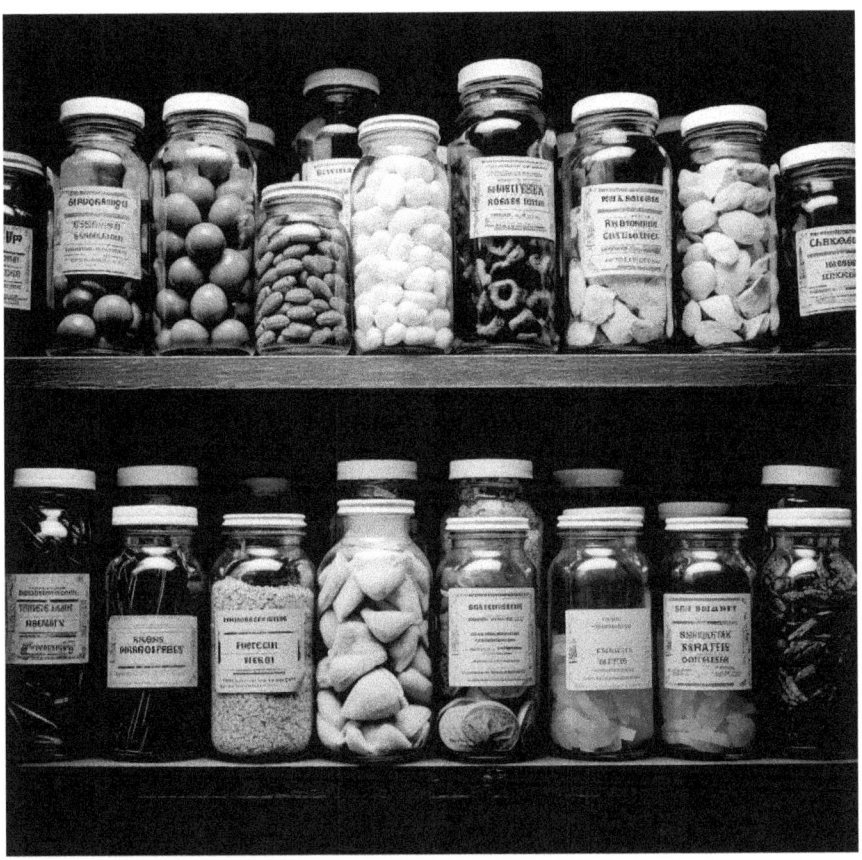

Vitamin D: Choose vitamin D capsules or tablets for bone health and immune support. Dosages vary but typically range from 600-2,000 IU daily.

Calcium: Calcium tablets are suitable for stockpiling and contribute to bone health. Adults usually require 1,000-1,200 mg per day.

Iron: Iron tablets or capsules can be essential, especially for those at risk of anemia during an emergency. Dosages vary, but typical recommendations range from 18-27 mg per day.

Magnesium: Magnesium is an essential mineral that plays a multitude of roles in maintaining our overall health. It's a cofactor for hundreds of enzymatic reactions in the body, contributing to processes like muscle function, nerve function, and energy production. Here are some compelling reasons why magnesium varieties should be part of your evolving emergency stockpile:

Magnesium Citrate: This is one of the most bioavailable forms of magnesium, making it effective for a wide range of applications such as regulating blood pressure, helping eliminate certain kidney stones, and muscle and nerve relaxation.

Magnesium Glycinate: It's a gentle form of magnesium that is well-absorbed and less likely to cause digestive discomfort. It's an excellent option for those with sensitive stomachs.

Magnesium Oxide: While less absorbable, magnesium oxide can still be valuable, especially for its laxative effects, which can be useful for digestive health.

Magnesium Chloride: This form of magnesium is often used for topical applications, such as in Epsom salt baths, but it can also be taken orally. It's beneficial for muscle relaxation.

Magnesium Sulfate: Epsom salt, or magnesium sulfate, is a versatile addition to your stockpile. It can be used both for oral supplementation and in baths for relaxation and muscle relief.

Spices and Flavor for Your Prepper Pantry

Spices and flavorings are often overlooked in prepper pantries, yet they are crucial for improving the taste and increasing morale at supper time, especially during long-term emergencies. These flavor-enhancing items can make your stockpile more versatile and enjoyable. Also keep in mind these spices are for the stockpile, not necessarily for your primary pantry. So many of these spices should be held as back-up for the primary container. Here are some considerations for when choosing flavors and then a comprehensive list of essential spices and flavorings:

Considerations:

Long Shelf Life: When choosing spices and flavorings for your prepper pantry, prioritize those with a long shelf life. Opt for dried herbs, spices, and other seasonings that remain potent for extended periods.

Variety: Ensure you have a variety of spices and seasonings to add depth and versatility to your meals. Different flavors can break the monotony of a limited stockpile menu.

Condiments: Include condiments like ketchup, mustard, mayonnaise, vinegar, and hot sauce for added flavor and variety. These items can be essential for making plain dishes more enjoyable.

Bouillon and Soup Bases: Bouillon cubes or granules and soup bases can add depth to soups and stews. They are shelf-stable and their compact size makes them space-efficient. They will provide culinary versatility and can be used as a base for many flavorful broths.

Essential Spices and Flavorings

Salt: Iodized salt, kosher salt, and sea salt are essential for seasoning and preserving food. This is spice #1 on the spice list for sure as it has so many uses in your home.

Black Pepper: Whole peppercorns or ground black pepper can add depth to a wide range of dishes.

Garlic Powder: Dried garlic powder is a versatile seasoning that adds a robust flavor to many dishes.

Onion Powder: Like garlic powder, onion powder can be used in a variety of recipes to add depth of flavor.

Paprika: Paprika comes in various varieties, including sweet, smoked, and hot, to suit different tastes and recipes.

Cayenne Pepper: A pinch of cayenne pepper can add heat and flavor to your meals.

Cumin: Ground cumin is excellent for seasoning chili, tacos, and other dishes.

Dried Oregano: Dried oregano is a staple in Mediterranean and Italian cuisine.

Dried Basil: Basil can be used in sauces, soups, and many Italian dishes.

Thyme: Dried thyme is perfect for adding a savory and earthy flavor to your recipes.

Rosemary: Rosemary adds a unique, pine-like flavor to dishes and is great for roasting meats.

Cinnamon: Cinnamon can be used in both sweet and savory dishes, including desserts and curries.

Nutmeg: Ground nutmeg is a versatile spice that compliments both sweet and savory recipes.

Curry Powder: Curry powder adds a complex blend of flavors to your dishes.

Dried Mustard: Dried mustard can be used to create a variety of condiments, dressings, and flavorings.

Red Pepper Flakes: These flakes are perfect for adding heat and spice to your meals.

Soy Sauce: Soy sauce is an excellent condiment for flavoring rice, stir-fries, and more.

Honey: Honey can be used as a natural sweetener and flavor enhancer in both sweet and savory dishes.

Vinegar: Vinegar can add acidity and brightness to your recipes. White, apple cider, and balsamic vinegar are versatile options.

Bouillon Cubes: These are excellent for making flavorful broths for soups and stews.

Hot Sauce: Hot sauce can add heat and flavor to a wide range of dishes.

Worcestershire Sauce: This sauce adds depth and umami to various recipes.

Sesame Oil: A small amount of sesame oil can add a distinctive flavor to stir-fries and Asian-inspired dishes.

To boost morale and add variety to your meals, include a selection of spices, herbs, and flavorings in your stockpile. These not only enhance taste but also provide potential health benefits.

Case Study: A Family's Journey to Good Health

The Allen family, faced with an extended emergency situation, maintained their health through a well-balanced stockpile. Their pantry included a variety of shelf-stable items representing key food groups. By supplementing with vitamins and minerals, they ensured that their nutritional needs were met during an extended power outage during a blizzard in 2022. Their story serves as a testament to the importance of nutrition in preparedness and the positive impact it can have on a family's health and well-being during crises.

Addressing Specific Dietary Considerations

When stockpiling for your family, it's crucial to account for individual dietary needs, such as restrictions and pre-existing health conditions.

Here's a comprehensive guide on how to accommodate these unique needs:

Lactose Intolerance: Opt for lactose-free dairy alternatives like almond or soy milk, and choose lactose-free dried dairy products for your stockpile.

Celiac Disease: Include gluten-free grains like rice, quinoa, and certified gluten-free pasta in your stockpile. Verify the gluten-free certification of your chosen products.

Diabetes: Store low-sugar, high-fiber foods like canned vegetables, whole grains, and lean proteins. Focus on complex carbohydrates and monitor carbohydrate intake during meal preparation.

Tree Nut Allergies: Avoid tree nuts and select nut-free protein sources like legumes and seeds. Check labels for potential cross-contamination with tree nuts.

Anemia: Prioritize iron-rich foods such as fortified cereals, lean meats, beans, and dark leafy greens in your stockpile. Ensure your iron sources are shelf-stable and accessible.

Egg Allergies: Substitute eggs with egg replacers or use alternatives like chia seeds or applesauce in your baking. When stocking up on baking essentials, make sure to choose egg substitutes that are safe for those with egg allergies.

Shellfish Allergies: To avoid allergic reactions, ensure that your stockpile does not include shellfish-based foods. Opt for alternative protein sources like beans, lentils, or canned fish like tuna or salmon, which do not pose the same allergen risks.

Hypertension (High Blood Pressure): High blood pressure requires a low-sodium diet. Stock low-sodium canned vegetables, and be mindful of salt in other food items. Also, select shelf-stable whole grains and lean proteins.

Pregnancy and Infant Nutrition: If you have an infant or are pregnant, your stockpile should include formula or breast milk alternatives, as well as baby food. Stock prenatal vitamins for expecting mothers to ensure they receive necessary prenatal nutrition.

Specialized Dietary Preferences: Accommodate any specialized dietary preferences within your family, such as vegetarian, vegan, or paleo diets. Ensure your stockpile accommodates these choices by including suitable foods that meet the family's nutritional requirements.

Pet Allergies: If you have family members with pet allergies, make sure that no pet allergens are present in your stockpile. Use a dedicated space and containers to store pet food, separate from your family's emergency supplies.

In the unpredictable world of emergency preparedness, nutritional balance and variety are not just ideals but practical necessities. By meticulously selecting and maintaining a diverse range of foods, supplementing with vitamins and minerals, and addressing specific dietary considerations for various health conditions, you are ensuring your family's well-being in good and bad times. Speaking of bad times, this next section will briefly discuss various forms of catastrophes your family may face, and provide further compelling reasons you should improve your food stockpile at home.

Catastrophes and Challenges

Different types of catastrophes pose unique safety challenges, and being prepared for these challenges is crucial. Historical context of disasters provides valuable insights into the importance of food stockpiling in various scenarios, let's take a closer look:

Natural Disasters: Natural disasters like hurricanes, earthquakes, floods, and wildfires can disrupt supply chains and make it difficult to access food. In the event of a major catastrophe, it's estimated that up to 95% of critical infrastructure could be affected, causing disruptions in the food supply chain. Food stockpiles become essential when stores are inaccessible. Consider the devastating impact of Hurricane Katrina, which left communities isolated without food or clean water for days. A well-planned stockpile can be the difference between survival and suffering. If you properly stockpile survival gear as well for your family, living near hurricane areas, these emergency items could be the difference between life and death.

Economic Crises: Economic downturns can lead to job losses, financial instability, and a scarcity of resources. A well-prepared stockpile acts as a financial safety net, reducing the strain on family resources. During times of economic crisis, stockpiling can help families reduce their expenses and provide food security even when finances are uncertain. During the great toilet paper shortage during the pandemic year 2020, my family rested easy when visiting the loo as we were well stocked!

Man-Made Events: Man-made disasters like power grid failures, civil unrest, or acts of terrorism can disrupt normal life. During these events, societal infrastructure can be compromised, making it difficult to access food through regular channels. Food stockpiling ensures self-reliance and minimizes your dependability on external resources when they may be unavailable or unsafe to access.

Personal Injury: Experiencing short-term or long-term disability due to injury significantly impacts one's ability to perform daily tasks, including shopping or cooking. A prepper pantry becomes essential in these situations as it ensures immediate access to food without relying on regular shopping trips or external assistance. For short-term disabilities, having a stocked pantry means having meals readily available, reducing the physical strain of preparing food while recovering.

In cases of long-term disability, a prepper pantry acts as a crucial resource hub, providing sustenance during extended periods of limited mobility or income. It allows individuals to maintain their nutritional needs without relying solely on outside help or delivery services, preserving a sense of autonomy and independence.

THE IMPORTANCE OF A 90-DAY SURVIVAL FOOD STOCKPILE

A 90-day survival food stockpile is a substantial resource, offering an extended safety net for your family during a catastrophe. The American Red Cross recommends that every household have a three-day supply of food and water. However, in more severe crises, such as extended power outages or natural disasters, a 90-day supply provides a substantial safety margin. This section explores many of the advantages of having such a stockpile in your home.

Extended Resilience: A 90-day supply ensures your family has enough food to sustain them while waiting for aid or normalcy to return. The average response time for emergency services during a disaster can be 48-72 hours, under-lining the importance of self-sufficiency. This extended resilience can make the difference between a short-term inconvenience and a long-term crisis.

Reduced Stress and Anxiety: Having an ample stockpile alleviates the anxiety of finding food during a crisis. It reduces the strain on your family's well-being and allows you to focus on other essential aspects of survival.

Nutritional Variety: With a 90-day stockpile, you can include a more extensive variety of foods, which contributes to better health during a crisis. A balanced diet minimizes the risk of nutrient deficiencies and their associated health problems.

Independence: A larger stockpile promotes self-reliance and reduces dependence on external resources. It empowers your family to meet its nutritional needs without relying on potentially overwhelmed relief efforts or supply chains during a disaster.

Coping with Prolonged Disruptions: During more prolonged disruptions, such as extended power outages or situations where normal food supplies are cut off, a 90-day stockpile becomes invaluable. During a power outage, refrigerated food can spoil within 4 hours, while a stocked pantry can last months. It ensures that your family has the necessary resources to endure extended challenges.

Investment in Security: While building a 90-day stockpile can be expensive initially, consider it as an investment in your family's security. You are essentially prepaying for food security during a crisis, which can significantly reduce the financial strain and uncertainty associated with unexpected emergencies. A simple strategy may be to buy double of a certain item every grocery trip. If you need black beans for your taco recipe that week, don't buy one can, buy two. Or better yet buy a Costco case and save it for your pantry.

Cost Spreading: Instead of purchasing all the items at once, you can gradually build your stockpile over time. By allocating a small portion of your budget to preparedness each month, the financial burden becomes more manageable. This gradual approach minimizes the impact on your finances and allows you to take advantage of sales and discounts.

Long-Term Savings: Consider the long-term savings of buying non-perishable items in bulk when they are on sale or when prices are low. You can potentially save money compared to buying smaller quantities at higher prices during an emergency. Your investment in a stockpile can pay off in the form of reduced grocery bills over time.

Optimized Storage Solutions: Make use of creative storage solutions to maximize space utilization. Utilize under-bed storage containers, vertical shelving units, and wall-mounted storage racks. By optimizing your available space, you can create a functional stockpile even in smaller homes or apartments.

Pantry Organization: Reorganize your pantry to accommodate stockpiled items. Many households have underutilized pantry space. By reorganizing and dedicating pantry shelves to your stockpile, you can make efficient use of existing storage.

Establish a System: Create a system for rotation. Use labels with purchase dates on your food items, so it's easy to identify which items need to be used first. Organize your stock-pile with older items at the front and newer ones at the back. By establishing a rotation system, you can efficiently manage your stockpile without wastage.

Alternate Storage Locations: Consider using alternate storage locations, such as your basement, garage, or even a rented storage unit, if space in your home is extremely limited. While this may incur an additional cost, it's a solution that can significantly expand your storage capacity.

Regular Inventory Checks: Schedule regular inventory checks. Set aside time every few months to review your stockpile. This practice helps you identify items that are nearing their expiration dates, allowing you to plan meals around these items or donate them to reduce waste.

Cooking from Stockpile: Incorporate meals using your stockpile items into your regular cooking routine. This not only helps with rotation but also keeps your family accustomed to the foods in your stockpile, ensuring that they will be comfortable eating these items during an emergency.

By considering a prepper pantry as a "serenity guarantee" project, and the initial cost as an investment, it will allow you to optimize your existing storage spaces and establish a rotation system. With this in mind, you can effectively address any challenges associated with maintaining a 90-day survival food stockpile. As seen above, the benefits surpass the drawbacks in establishing or growing your food stockpile. These proactive approaches will make your stockpile more practical, manageable, and cost-effective.

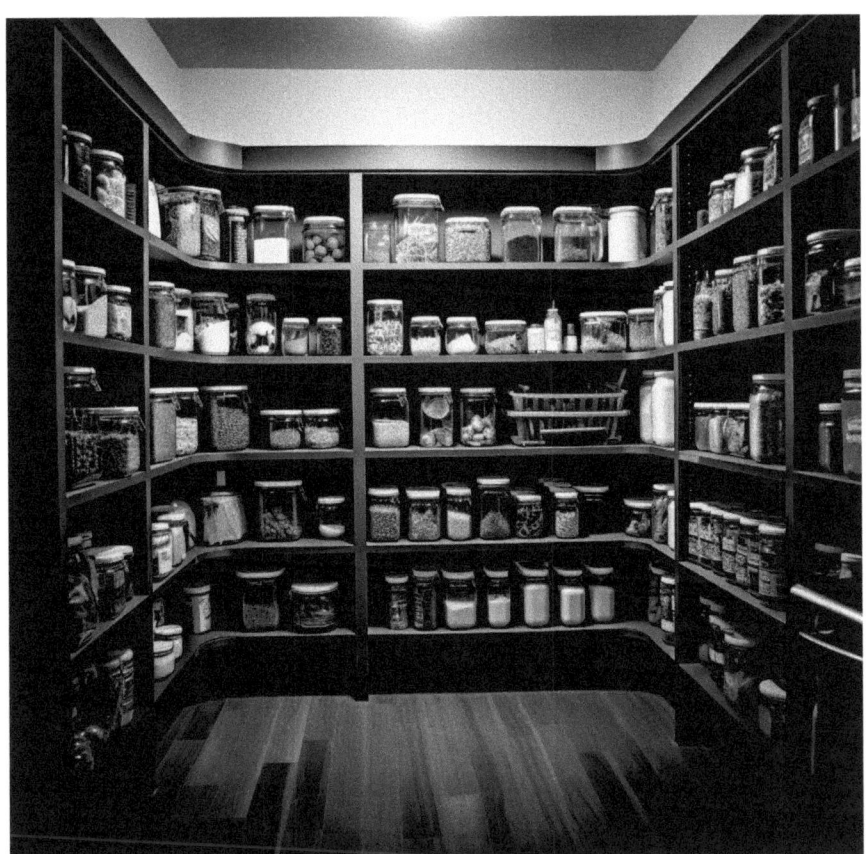

SETTING REALISTIC GOALS

Setting realistic goals is pivotal in your journey toward preparedness.

Here's a more detailed checklist to guide your efforts:

Get Your Home Ready for 2 Weeks of Self-Reliance: Start with a two-week supply of food, water, and essential supplies. This initial goal is achievable and provides a foundation for further preparedness. It also should not break the bank! Consider involving your family in meal planning and teaching them how to use the stored items so that they are actively engaged in the preparedness process. In a world where unexpected challenges can arise, being prepared is not merely an option; it is a responsibility, a commitment to resilience, and a testament to your dedication to the safety and security of those you hold dear.

Be Able to Bug-Out at a Moment's Notice: Develop a bug-out bag (BOB) for each family member, with essential items like food, water, clothing, mylar sleeping bag, flashlight, fire starter, and important documents. Ensure your family is familiar with its contents and how to use them. Regularly review and update your bug-out bag to account for changing needs and seasonal considerations, ensuring it remains a reliable resource. I just spent a Sunday afternoon with my youngest daughter, who volunteered to help, go through our families BOB's and restock where needed. It was quality time with my baby girl, we had fun, and it checked off an important "to do" list item for our entire family!

Prepare for Emergencies Away from Home with a "Get-Home Bag": Having a get-home bag (GHB) in your vehicle or at work can be invaluable. Ensure it contains the essentials you might need to safely return home during an emergency. Familiarize your family with the concept of a get-home bag and the importance of its contents, so they are prepared even when away from home. It is prudent to explore multiple commuting routes from your workplace to your residence using a physical map. This precaution becomes particularly relevant in scenarios where the power grid fails, rendering GPS navigation unavailable. Expert tip, my GHB items account for land travel 40 miles from my office to my home if necessary (think boots, mylar sleeping bag, 72-hrs worth of food and water, fire starter, and a weapon). You may not require these items if you travel in a 5 mile radius from home, I'm just stating my situation. Furthermore, it is advisable to cultivate heightened situational awareness during your daily commutes, envisioning a hypothetical situation where you may need to traverse the distance on foot, making your way back to your family. This practice not only prepares you for unforeseen circumstances but also adds an element of mindfulness to your daily routines.

Learn Core Survival Skills: Acquire basic survival skills such as first aid, fire-starting, navigation, and emergency communication. These skills are foundational for survival and should be practiced regularly. If power is out, igniting a fire for cooking or boiling water. The difference lies between a night endured hungry and cold, versus a night embraced with a warm meal and comfort for sleep. Learn these skills now, don't put this off to "figure out" when the situation arises. When a catastrophe strikes, numerous pressing matters arise, especially when responsibilities exist for you to also help other family members. Managing basic tasks becomes challenging in a worst-case scenario, and there's a risk of struggling or failing to address even the most fundamental needs amidst the chaos. Absorb, rehearse, repeat—this cannot be emphasized sufficiently! Explore enrolling in courses or workshops now to expand your skill set. Encourage your family to participate as well, nurturing a shared knowledge base.

Practice with Your Gear: Familiarize yourself and your family with your survival gear, including cooking equipment, water purification tools, and emergency lighting. Regular practice ensures that you can use these items effectively during an emergency. Organize family "practice drills" to simulate emergency scenarios, which can help your loved ones become confident in using the equipment when it truly matters.

By understanding the core principles of food stockpiling, the psychology of preparedness, the value of a 90-day survival food stockpile, and setting realistic goals, you are better equipped to ensure your family's safety and well-being during a catastrophe. Preparedness isn't just about stockpiling; it's a holistic approach to self-reliance and resilience in the face of adversity.

As you continue on this path, remember that the goal is not just to survive but to thrive during adversity. Your commitment to preparedness serves as a testament to your dedication to the well-being of your family, and the strength of your community. The journey is as important as the destination, and the skills and knowledge you acquire will empower you to confront whatever challenges life may bring. Preparing now is an investment in your family's safety and well-being, and it ensures that you have the tools and the mindset to face an unpredictable future.

BUILDING YOUR 90-DAY SURVIVAL FOOD STOCKPILE: A FOUNDATION OF SECURITY

"Stockpiling food is like having insurance for your family's survival."

— CARLOS MACK

A SOBERING REALITY

In today's world, it's alarming to consider that 43% of American families are unprepared for disasters, lacking essential emergency supplies, including food and water, in their homes. This statistic from the Federal Emergency Management Agency (FEMA) underscores the urgent need for preparedness, education, and action from you. By proactively equipping your home, and your mindset, for emergency situations, you are taking a proactive stance toward safeguarding the well-being of yourself and your loved ones.

Determining Caloric and Nutritional Requirements

To build an effective 90-day survival food stockpile, it's crucial to begin with a clear understanding of the caloric and nutritional needs of each family member, from the young to the elderly. Calorie considerations can often be an overlooked aspect of stockpiling. Your food supply should not just sustain you, but provide enough energy to carry you through the crisis. The general guideline is to have at least 2,000 calories per day per person, which is the average daily caloric intake.

CALCULATING CALORIC NEEDS: UNDERSTANDING THE BASICS

Ensuring that your stockpile provides sufficient calories for each family member is the first step here. This calculation, however, is not one-size-fits-all and requires consideration of several factors.

To accurately assess daily caloric requirements for each person in your household, you must account for some variables. These can include age, sex, activity level, and underlying health conditions. For instance, a growing child will require fewer calories than an active adult, and a pregnant woman's needs will significantly differ from those of an elderly family member. To further illustrate the importance of this, let's delve into some key statistics and guidelines:

Age: Children generally require fewer calories than adults due to their smaller size and lower activity levels. For example, a moderately active 8-year-old boy might need around 1,600 to 2,200 calories per day, while an active adult male could require 2,200 to 3,200 calories daily.

Sex: Gender plays a significant role in caloric requirements. On average, men tend to need more calories than women. For example, a sedentary adult woman might require around 1,800 to 2,200 calories per day, while a sedentary adult man could need 2,200 to 2,800 calories daily.

Activity Level: The level of physical activity is a crucial factor. An active lifestyle demands more calories to fuel physical exertion. A moderately active person might require 10% to 30% more calories than a sedentary individual.

Underlying Health Conditions: Medical conditions such as diabetes, heart disease, or metabolic disorders can impact nutritional needs. For instance, in diabetes, there might be impaired insulin function leading to difficulties in regulating blood sugar levels. Hence, caloric intake and the types of nutrients consumed need to be carefully monitored to avoid spikes or drops in blood sugar. Or those with heart disease may have restrictions on sodium and fluid intake to manage their condition. Some medications used to manage these conditions can affect nutrient absorption or utilization as well. It's essential to consider these factors when calculating caloric requirements.

While a general guideline is to aim for 2,000 calories per day per person, this is a broad estimate that might not suit everyone's needs. Therefore, it's advisable to calculate the specific requirements for each family member, taking into account their individual circumstances. Calculating the calorie content of your stored food items and ensuring that you meet your family's daily caloric needs is crucial. This understanding ensures that your stockpile is not just a collection of random food items but a carefully planned resource for survival.

SOURCING SURVIVAL FOODS AND ESTABLISHING SELF-SUFFICIENCY MEASURES

Types of Survival Foods: A Comprehensive Guide to Preserving

When building your prepper pantry, understanding the different types of survival foods is essential. Each category has its advantages, and knowing when to use them is crucial for maintaining a well-balanced stockpile. In this section, we'll delve into the four primary categories of survival foods and explore their characteristics in short detail.

In the realm of preserving food through dehydrating, canning, freeze drying, and jerky making, entire libraries of knowledge reside within books, podcasts, and websites dedicated to each method. However, in this chapter, I offer a brief glimpse into these techniques, recognizing their vast complexity and depth.

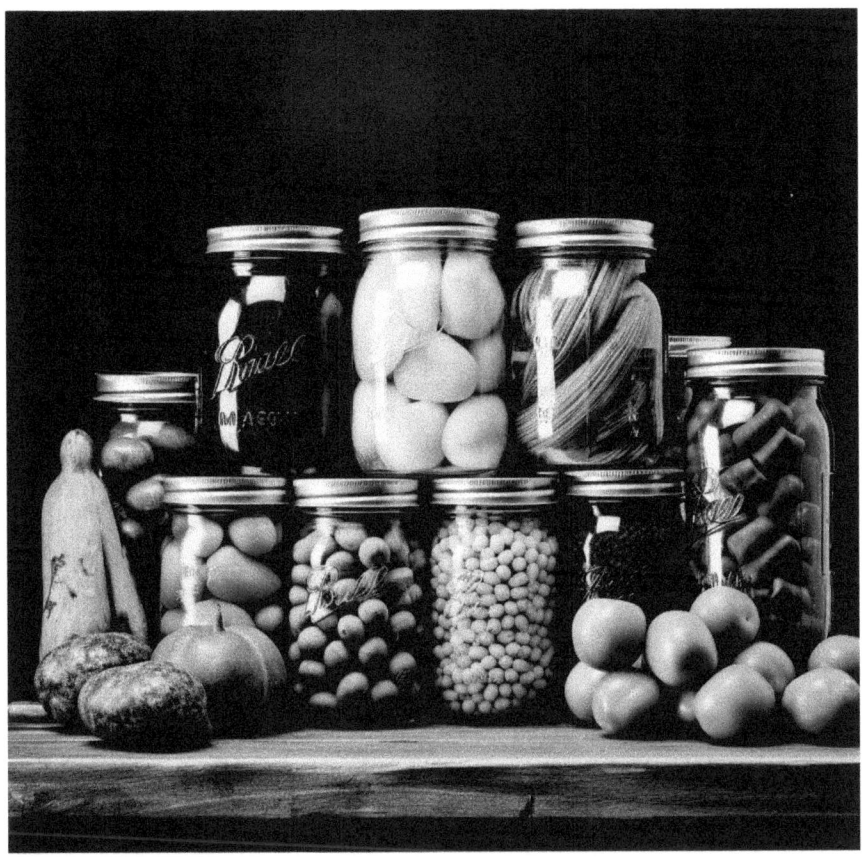

Consider this section a preliminary introduction, a stepping stone toward understanding these preservation methods. It is advisable, after experimenting and discovering what aligns best with your family's needs, to seek further guidance from these extensive resources. Delving deeper into these practices, informed by experience and personal preferences, can yield invaluable insights and mastery.

Dehydrated Foods: Preserving Nutrition Through Dehydration

Dehydrating is an excellent way to remove moisture from fruits, vegetables, and herbs. Removing moisture is a sound way to prevent the growth of microorganisms and bacteria. As a result, these foods can last for years, making them an excellent addition to your stockpile.

I've touched on dehydrating in several sections in the book as it is a vital element to so many different aspects of a thriving prepper pantry. To dehydrate food, you will need a dehydrator or an oven with a low-temperature setting. Ensure the food is sliced into uniform pieces for even drying. Dehydrated foods are a popular choice among preppers due to their lightweight nature and extended shelf life. Dehydrated foods come in various forms, including fruits, vegetables, and complete meals in pouches. They maintain much of their original nutritional value, as the dehydration process primarily affects water content. While they might not be as flavorful as fresh alternatives, they remain a dependable source of essential vitamins and minerals during an emergency.

Equipment needed:

Food dehydrator
Fresh fruits or vegetables

Steps:

- Wash and prepare the fruits or vegetables by slicing them uniformly for even drying.
- Arrange the slices on the dehydrator trays, leaving space between each piece for proper air circulation.
- Set the dehydrator to the appropriate temperature and duration based on the food being dehydrated. Fruits generally dry at lower temperatures (around 135°F/57°C), while vegetables might require higher temperatures.
- Allow the dehydrator to run until the food is fully dried. Check regularly to monitor progress.
- Once dried, let the food cool completely before storing it in airtight containers or vacuum-sealed bags. Properly dried foods should be brittle and without moisture.

Dehydrating Food Safely:

Cleanliness: Begin with a clean working environment. Sanitize all equipment, trays, and tools before use to prevent the transfer of bacteria to your food.

Proper Preparation: Wash fruits, vegetables, and herbs thoroughly before dehydrating. Remove any damaged or spoiled parts to prevent mold growth.

Uniform Slicing: Cut your produce into uniform pieces to ensure consistent drying. This helps prevent under-drying or over-drying, which can lead to spoilage.

Temperature Control: Set the dehydrator at the recommended temperature for each type of food. Different foods require specific temperatures for safe preservation.

Monitoring: Regularly check the progress of your dehydrating food. It should be dry to the touch but still pliable. Over-drying can reduce flavor and nutritional value.

Cooling and Storage: Let the dehydrated items cool to room temperature before storing. Store them in airtight containers in a cool, dark place to prevent moisture absorption and spoilage.

Canning Foods: Convenience Meets Reliability

Canning goods have long been a staple in prepper pantries, thanks to their convenience and stable shelf life. The World Health Organization recommends storing at least 400 pounds of food per person to ensure survival during extended emergencies, and canning will bring you closer to that desired weight in food. In my pantry, I employ different canning methods such as water bath canning, pressure canning, and pickling to preserve a variety of foods for long-term storage. The canning process involves sealing food in an airtight container, effectively preventing spoilage. Canned foods can last for several years, and with proper rotation, you can maintain their freshness. Let's look at pressure canning more in-depth:

Equipment needed:

Pressure canner or water bath canner
Glass canning jars with lids and bands
Fresh produce or other ingredients for canning
Jar lifter, funnel, and other canning tools

Steps:

- Prepare the food according to a trusted canning recipe. This might involve blanching, cooking, or treating the ingredients as required.
- Sterilize the canning jars, lids, and bands by boiling them or using the sanitize cycle on a dishwasher.
- Fill the jars with the prepared food using a canning funnel, leaving the appropriate headspace as specified in the recipe.
- Wipe the jar rims clean, place the lids and bands on the jars, and tighten them finger-tight.
- Process the jars in a pressure canner or water bath canner according to the recipe and guidelines for the specific food being canned.

- Once processed, carefully remove the jars using a jar lifter and place them on a towel to cool. Listen for the distinctive "pop" of the lids sealing as they cool.

Canning Food Safely:

Hygiene is Key: Maintain meticulous cleanliness. Sterilize jars, lids, and equipment before use to prevent contamination and spoilage.

Follow Tested Recipes: Use reliable and tested canning recipes from trusted sources like USDA or reputable canning guides. Follow recipes precisely to ensure safe canning methods and proper processing times.

Mind Altitude and Pressure: Adjust canning times and pressures based on your altitude. High altitudes require increased processing times or pressures for safe canning.

Check for Seals: After canning, check for sealed jars. Press the lid; if it doesn't flex or make a popping sound, the jar is sealed. Store unsealed jars in the fridge or reprocess them.

Label and Rotate Stock: Label jars with contents and date canned. Rotate stock regularly, using older items first to maintain freshness.

Storage and Inspection: Store canned goods in a cool, dark place. Regularly inspect cans for signs of spoilage, including bulging lids, leakage, off-odors, or mold growth.

Know When to Discard: If there's any doubt about the safety of canned goods, discard them. Never taste suspicious food; it's better to be safe than sorry when it comes to canned food safety.

One of the benefits of canned foods is their versatility. From vegetables and fruits to meats and soups, you can find a wide array of options. However, it's crucial to pay attention to expiration dates and rotate your canned items regularly. Doing so ensures that you always have fresh, nutritious options on hand when needed.

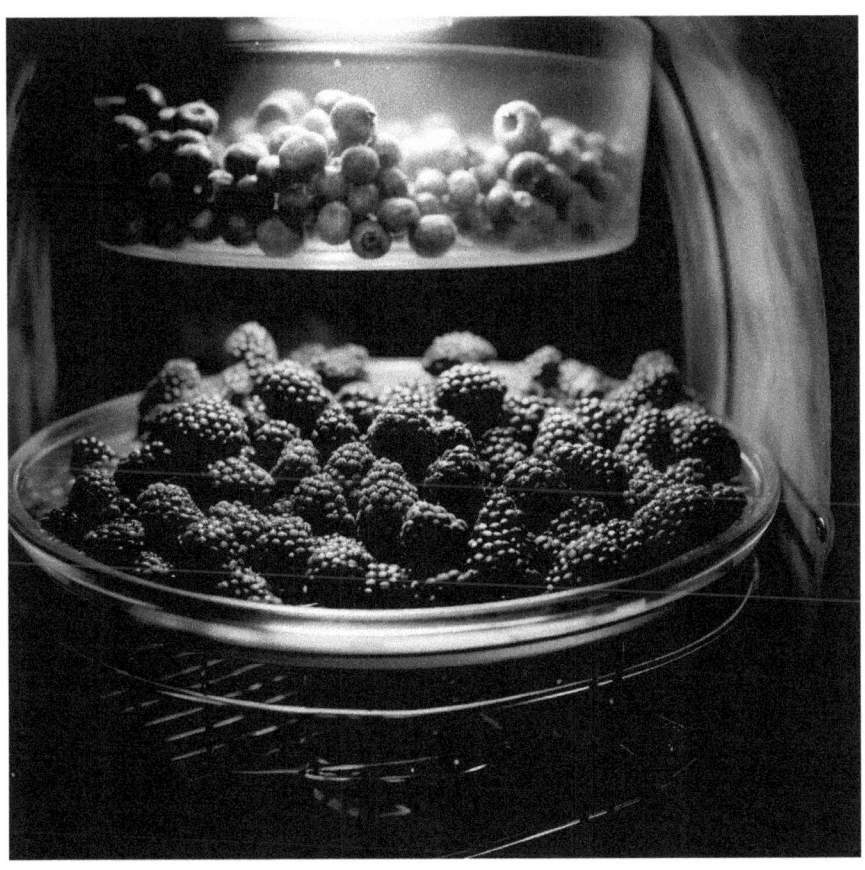

Freeze-Dried Foods: Lightweight and Nutrient-Packed

Freeze-dried foods are celebrated for their lightweight nature, exceptional nutritional content, and extended shelf life. Freeze drying takes preservation a step further by freezing food and then slowly removing the ice, leaving behind a dried product. This method retains the food's original shape, color, flavor, and nutritional value. The result is a lightweight, crunchy product.

These foods can last for decades, and their lightweight nature makes them an excellent choice for bug-out bags and portable emergency kits. When rehydrated, freeze-dried meals regain their original taste, making them a delicious and nutritious option during crises. They are available in various forms, from individual ingredients like fruits and vegetables to complete meals in pouches. To freeze dry, you'll need a freeze dryer, which is an investment, but it offers unmatched quality and longevity in preserved food. When using a freeze dryer, follow the manufacturer's guidelines for different foods to ensure the best results.

Equipment needed:

Freeze dryer machine
Fresh foods or ingredients

Steps:

- Prepare the food by slicing or portioning it appropriately for freeze-drying.
- Arrange the food on the trays of the freeze dryer, ensuring proper spacing for even drying.
- Place the trays in the freeze dryer and start the machine. The freeze dryer will freeze the food and then slowly reduce the pressure, allowing the frozen water to evaporate.
- The process can take several hours or even days, depending on the food and the freeze dryer's capacity.
- Once the food is freeze-dried, remove it from the machine. It should be dry, lightweight, and crisp.
- Store the freeze-dried food in airtight containers or Mylar bags with oxygen absorbers to maintain its quality and shelf life.

Freezing Food Safely:

Preparation: Ensure that food going into the freezer is in the best possible condition. Blanch vegetables before freezing to preserve flavor, color, and nutritional value.

Packaging: Use airtight, moisture-proof containers or freezer bags to prevent freezer burn. Remove as much air as possible to maintain food quality.

Labeling: Clearly label all frozen items with the date of freezing to help with rotation and to ensure the oldest items are used first.

Safe Temperatures: Keep your freezer at or below 0°F (-18°C) to prevent bacterial growth. Invest in a freezer thermometer to monitor the temperature.

Thawing: Thaw frozen food in the refrigerator or, if necessary, under cold running water. Never leave food at room temperature for extended periods, as this promotes bacterial growth.

Refreezing: It's generally safe to refreeze food that has been thawed in the refrigerator. However, avoid repeated thawing and freezing, as this can impact quality.

JERKY JOURNEY: TRANSFORMING MEAT INTO IRRESISTIBLE CHEWY GOODNESS!

Jerky making is a popular method for preserving meat. It involves marinating thin strips of meat and then drying them to remove moisture. This process helps prevent spoilage while creating a tasty protein source. A dehydrator or an oven with low-temperature settings is ideal for making jerky. Proper storage in airtight containers is crucial to maintain its quality.

Making jerky requires minimal equipment and a few straight-forward steps. Here's what you'll need and the basic process:

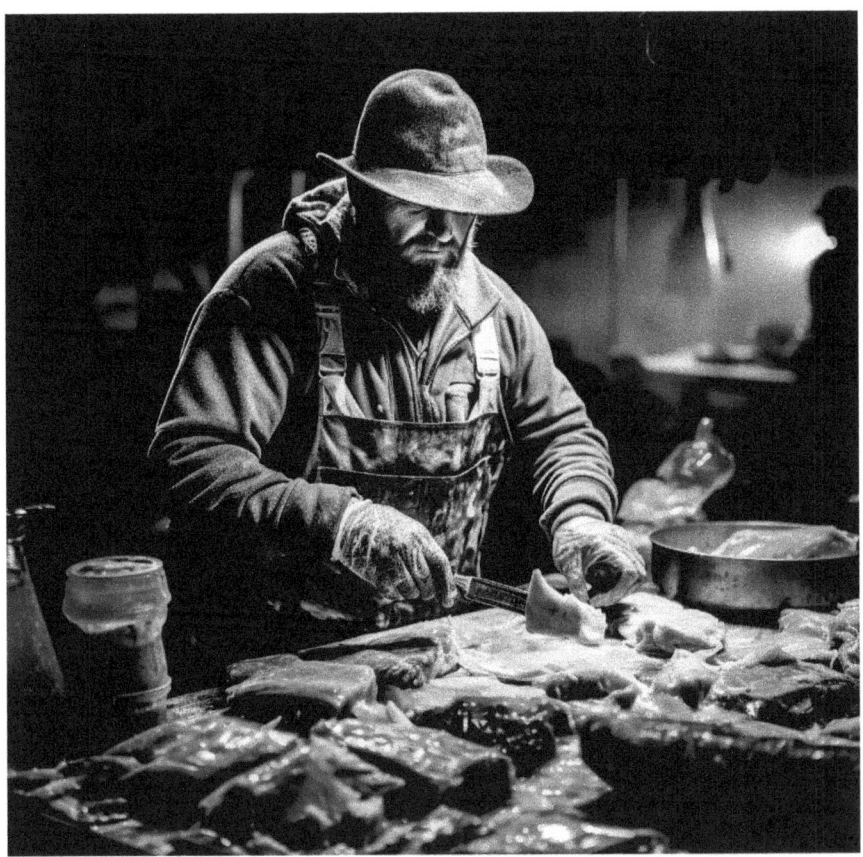

Equipment Needed:

Dehydrator or Oven: Dehydrators offer consistent low heat ideal for drying jerky, but ovens set to low temperatures can work too.

Sharp Knife: For slicing meat into thin strips.

Cutting Board: To prepare and slice the meat.

Marinade Ingredients: For flavoring (ingredients vary based on preference).
Plastic or Glass Container: To marinate the meat.
Paper Towels: For patting dry the meat before drying.

Steps:

- Choose lean cuts like beef (flank steak, sirloin, or round), venison, or poultry. Trim excess fat and slice against the grain into thin strips (around 1/4 inch thick).
- Prepare a marinade using ingredients like soy sauce, Worcestershire sauce, liquid smoke, spices, or sugar. Place the meat strips in a plastic or glass container, cover with the marinade, and refrigerate for at least 6-24 hours.
- Remove the meat from the marinade and pat it dry with paper towels to remove excess moisture.
- Arrange the meat strips on dehydrator trays or oven racks, leaving space between pieces for air circulation. Set the dehydrator to around 145°F (63°C) or the oven to its lowest setting and prop the door open slightly to allow moisture to escape. Dry the jerky for 4-12 hours until it reaches your desired consistency (it should bend without breaking).
- Once dried, let the jerky cool completely. If any moisture remains, blot it with paper towels. Store in

airtight containers or vacuum-sealed bags for longer shelf life.

Making Jerky Safely:

Food Safety Practices: Follow general food safety guidelines for handling meat, including proper handwashing, sanitization, and safe storage practices, to prevent foodborne illnesses.

Meat Selection: Choose lean meats and trim visible fat. Fat can become rancid during storage and reduce shelf life.

Proper Preparation: Use clean utensils, cutting boards, and hands while handling raw meat. Sanitize equipment and surfaces before and after use to prevent cross-contamination.

Thin and Even Slicing: Slice meat into uniform thickness (around 1/4 inch) for even drying. Thicker slices might not dry properly and could harbor bacteria.

Marinade and Refrigeration: Marinate meat in the refrigerator, not at room temperature, to prevent bacterial growth. Always discard leftover marinade that's been in contact with raw meat.

Temperature Control: Ensure meat reaches a safe temperature during drying to destroy harmful bacteria. The dehydrator or oven should maintain a consistent temperature of at least 160°F (71°C) to kill pathogens.

Remember to follow food safety guidelines and ensure the jerky reaches a safe internal temperature to kill bacteria during the drying process. If using an oven, periodically check for doneness to prevent over-drying.

By including items from each of these categories, you ensure that your stockpile is not only well-balanced, but also adaptable to various emergency scenarios. Food preservation techniques are essential for self-sufficiency. They extend the shelf life of food, reducing waste and ensuring you have a steady supply of nourishment. When it comes to the preservation techniques mentioned earlier, feel free to share any tweaks or family recipes you have that might improve the instructions or equipment used for these methods. Your passed-down wisdom might offer a better way to approach one of these preservation techniques. In fact, I'd love to hear from you on my Facebook page "lighthouse survival" or comment or email me on my website: www.lighthousesurvival.net. I absolutely love messaging with my fans on how they do what they do. There is no "one-size-fits-all" way to prep, so your fresh ideas and feedback are welcome here! Regarding food preservation, I offered beginner-friendly guidelines, but there's a wealth of knowledge waiting for you in specialized courses or books solely dedicated to these preservation techniques. You can explore these resources at your own pace to delve deeper into the subject. So whether you're sheltering in place or on the move, these preserved survival foods will be your reliable sources of nutrition and sustenance during challenging times.

NON-PERISHABLE STAPLES: THE BUILDING BLOCKS OF SURVIVAL MEALS

Non-perishable staples serve as the foundation of your prepper pantry. These staple items, including pasta, rice, flour, and sugar. They are ingredients that are versatile, long-lasting, and essential for creating a variety of meals. These are the building blocks for countless recipes, ensuring that you can prepare satisfying and nutritious dishes during emergencies.

Pasta and rice, for example, are carbohydrate-rich staples that can serve as the base for various recipes. Flour is crucial for baking bread and making thickening agents for soups and stews. Sugar adds sweetness to beverages and desserts, providing comfort even in challenging times. Non-perishable staples are easy to store and have relatively long shelf lives, making them fundamental components of your stockpile. According to a FEMA report, 70% of all declared disasters involve some level of power outage, highlighting the need for non-perishable food storage.

MORE SHELF-STABLE FOODS THAT PROVIDE A WELL-ROUNDED NUTRITIONAL PROFILE

Your 90-day survival food stockpile should consist of a variety of shelf-stable foods that offer a balanced nutritional profile. I listed the "staples" for shelf-stable pantry foundations, these are extra credit items, for that nutritional punch your family will need. This ensures that every family member receives the nutrients they need to maintain health and strength, as well as variety, avoiding food boredom. Here is a detailed list of foods to consider for your pantry stash:

Chia Seeds: These tiny seeds are packed with omega-3 fatty acids, fiber, antioxidants, and protein. They can be added to smoothies, oatmeal, or used as a thickening agent in recipes.

Hemp Seeds: High in protein, omega-3s, and omega-6s, hemp seeds are a nutritious addition to the diet. They provide a complete source of protein and are rich in essential fatty acids.

Tahini: Made from ground sesame seeds, tahini is a good source of healthy fats, protein, and minerals like magnesium and calcium. It's versatile and can be used in dressings, sauces, or as a spread.

Nutritional Yeast: A great source of B vitamins, particularly B12 for vegans or vegetarians. It has a cheesy flavor and can be sprinkled on dishes as a topping or used to make dairy-free sauces.

Dried Seaweed: Seaweed, like nori, dulse, or kelp, is rich in vitamins (especially B12 in certain varieties), minerals like iodine, and antioxidants. It's a great addition to soups, salads, or used to wrap foods.

Canned or Dried Dairy: Evaporated milk, powdered milk, and cheese are dairy options that provide essential calcium for bone health and protein for muscle maintenance. These dairy items can be used in cooking, baking, or as a beverage. Powdered milk is a versatile choice as it has a longer shelf life compared to liquid milk.

Canned Soups and Stews: Canned soups and stews can be complete meals in themselves. They often contain a combination of proteins, vegetables, and carbohydrates, providing a well-rounded nutritional profile. Having a selection of these canned options in your pantry ensures that you have quick and convenient meal choices during emergencies.

Canned Fish: Beyond canned tuna, consider options like salmon or sardines. These fish choices are rich in omega-3 fatty acids, which are essential for heart and brain health. Including a variety of canned fish in your stockpile ensures a diverse source of protein and healthy fats.

Dried Fruits and Nuts: These options offer essential vitamins, minerals, and healthy fats. Dried fruits like raisins and apricots provide natural sweetness and a dose of energy, while nuts such as almonds and walnuts offer protein and healthy fats. They are excellent choices for on-the-go snacks or as additions to your meals.

Multivitamins: While your stockpile focuses on whole foods, including a supply of multivitamins is a wise choice. These supplements can help compensate for potential nutrient gaps that may occur during an emergency. Multivitamins ensure that your family receives a broad spectrum of essential vitamins and minerals for overall health and well-being.

With these detailed explanations, you can now confidently curate your prepper pantry, ensuring that it provides a comprehensive and balanced nutritional profile for your family during unforeseen challenges.

A well-rounded prepper pantry includes a diverse range of survival foods, each with its unique advantages. Dehydrated foods offer extended shelf life while preserving essential nutrients. Canned foods provide convenience and versatility. Non-perishable staples serve as the foundation for survival meals, and freeze-dried foods are lightweight and nutrient-packed.

Selecting and Sourcing Health Foods for Stockpiling

In the quest for an effective and balanced stockpile, it's prudent to consider healthy foods as an integral part of your preparedness strategy. These are the gems of nutrition - non-GMO, organic, and minimally processed options, renowned for their ability to sustain your well-being during trying times.

HEALTH FOODS: A COMMITMENT TO WELL-BEING

Non-GMO and Organic Foods: When it comes to health foods, these are the gold standard. Non-GMO and organic items are cultivated with minimal interference from genetic modification and harmful pesticides. The benefits of these choices extend beyond your personal health. By selecting non-GMO and organic options, you reduce the risk of potential health complications associated with GMOs and contribute to a more sustainable and environmentally responsible food production system.

Minimally Processed Foods: The allure of minimally processed foods lies in their purity. These items are intentionally kept simple, with fewer additives and preservatives. The result is a product with cleaner, healthier ingredients. By incorporating minimally processed foods into your stockpile, you ensure that you and your family have access to nutrition that is as close to its natural state as possible.

POSITIVES OF STOCKING HEALTH FOODS: NOURISHING THE BODY AND MIND

Enhanced Nutrition: Health foods are synonymous with superior nutrition. They are brimming with essential vitamins, minerals, and nutrients, providing your family with a healthier diet during emergencies. For instance, organic produce tends to have higher levels of certain antioxidants and micronutrients compared to their conventionally grown counterparts.

Peace of Mind: Stocking health foods is more than just a dietary choice; it's a commitment to a healthy lifestyle that remains unwavering even in the face of crises. Knowing that you have wholesome options in your pantry can bring peace of mind, offering solace during uncertain times. This sense of continuity with your regular diet can boost morale and mental resilience.

NEGATIVES OF STOCKING HEALTH FOODS: WEIGHING THE COSTS

Opting for health-conscious choices when assembling your stockpile, while commendable, is not without its trade-offs. Below, we delve into some of the factors to take into account when prioritizing well-being in your emergency food reserves.

Higher Cost: While the benefits of healthy foods are undeniable, they often come at a higher price point compared to their conventional counterparts. This price difference is a result of the more labor-intensive farming methods, certification costs, and lower yields associated with organic and non-GMO production. Consider this aspect when building your stockpile and balance it with your budget.

Shorter Shelf Life: Health foods typically have a shorter shelf life compared to heavily processed items laden with preservatives. The reduced use of additives and extended processing times can lead to a more limited storage duration. It's crucial to monitor expiration dates and regularly rotate these items to maintain their quality.

Availability: Finding organic or non-GMO versions of certain foods can be more challenging, depending on your location. While these items are increasingly available, their presence may still be limited in some areas. Keep this in mind as you plan your stockpile and be open to incorporating conventional items where necessary.

DIETARY PREFERENCES: A PERSONALIZED APPROACH

In the realm of preparedness, customization is key. Consider the dietary preferences and restrictions of your family members when building your 90-day survival food pantry. Whether your loved ones follow vegetarian, vegan, gluten-free, or other specific diets, ensure that your stockpile accommodates these choices.

Plant-Based Protein Sources: For vegetarians and vegans, plant-based protein sources are essential. These can include dried legumes, tofu, and plant-based protein powders.

Gluten-Free Grains: Those with gluten sensitivities should stock up on gluten-free grains such as rice, quinoa, and gluten-free flour to ensure that their dietary needs are met.

Specialized Products: If any family members have particular dietary requirements, be it due to allergies, intolerances, or personal choices, make sure your stockpile includes specialized products that cater to those needs. Look for items that align with these dietary preferences and restrictions.

By considering the positive and negative aspects of stocking healthy foods and accommodating dietary preferences, your stockpile becomes not just a source of sustenance, but a reflection of your family's unique needs and values. It serves as a testament to your dedication to their well-being, even in the face of adversity.

10 STEPS TO A WELL-STOCKED PANTRY

In the world of emergency preparedness, a well-stocked pantry stands as a cornerstone of resilience and self-reliance. It's a vital resource that ensures your family's nutritional needs are met during challenging times. While the idea of a prepper pantry might seem overwhelming at first, it's a journey that begins with small, manageable steps. Whether you're new to preparedness or a seasoned prepper, these ten steps will guide you in building a well-organized and well-stocked pantry that can serve as a reliable lifeline when needed.

Start Small: Begin by adding a few extra canned goods and non-perishable items to your weekly grocery shopping.

Plan Your Meals: Plan meals around the items in your stockpile to ensure they get used and replaced regularly.

Organize Regularly: Create a system for rotating food items, ensuring that older items are used first.

Label and Date: Label items with the purchase date to facilitate proper rotation.

Monitor Expiration Dates: Keep an eye on expiration dates and replace items as needed.

Include Essentials: Don't forget basics like salt, sugar, and cooking oil in your pantry.

Prioritize Water: Water is essential for survival, so ensure you have a reliable water supply.

Consider Special Diets: If you have dietary restrictions, stockpile accordingly.

Add Variety: Include a variety of foods to keep meals interesting during an emergency.

Educate Your Family: Teach your family about your stockpile and how to use the items within it.

The journey to a well-stocked pantry is not a sprint but a marathon, marked by careful planning and steady progress. With each step you take, you build a stronger foundation for your family's well-being during emergencies. By starting small, meal planning, organizing, and staying vigilant about expiration dates, you ensure that your pantry remains a source of comfort and sustenance. Remember to educate your family about its contents and use – knowledge that might prove invaluable during a crisis. A well-stocked pantry is more than a collection of goods; it's a symbol of your preparedness, your commitment to safety, and your dedication to protecting the ones you love.

Building a Stockpile on A Budget

While the initial cost of building a 90-day survival food stockpile can be a concern, there are practical ways to address budget constraints without compromising on preparedness.

Costs of Emergency Preparedness

It's worth noting that emergency preparedness does involve some costs. According to surveys, the budget for prepping in the United States varies widely, with some people spending as little as $50 per month and others investing hundreds of dollars each month.

PRACTICAL TIPS FOR STOCKPILING ON A BUDGET

To build a well-rounded stockpile without breaking the bank, consider these practical tips:

Set a Budget: Establish a monthly budget specifically for emergency preparedness. Even a small allocation can make a significant difference over time.

Buy in Bulk: Purchase items in bulk when they are on sale. Look for discounts, bulk bins, and online deals to get more for your money. A well-prepared pantry can save you up to

$500 annually by taking advantage of sales and buying in bulk.

Prioritize Essentials: Focus on acquiring essential items first, such as water, canned goods, and non-perishable staples. Gradually expand your stockpile to include other items.

Store-Brand Products: Store-brand or generic products are often more affordable and can be of comparable quality to name brands.

Coupon and Discount Apps: Utilize coupon and discount apps to save on groceries. Many apps offer digital coupons and cashback incentives.

Meal Planning: Plan meals around what you have in your stockpile to minimize food waste and save on groceries.

DIY Food Preservation: Learn food preservation techniques like canning, dehydrating, or freezing to extend the shelf life of fresh foods and reduce costs.

Rotate Items Efficiently: Implement a system to rotate items in your stockpile so that nothing goes to waste due to expiration.

Community Efforts: Consider collaborating with neighbors or friends to purchase items in bulk, share costs, and divide resources, making preparedness more affordable.

SUCCESS STORY - THE PETERSON FAMILY:

Meet the Peterson's, a budget-conscious family who successfully built an extensive stockpile without breaking the bank. They started by allocating a modest monthly budget to preparedness. By diligently purchasing items on sale, taking advantage of coupons, and bulk-buying during promotions, they accumulated an impressive stockpile over the years. The Peterson's focused on building a rotation system to minimize waste and prioritize essential items. Their efforts paid off when they experienced a prolonged power outage due to a severe storm. Their well-prepared pantry provided them with peace of mind and comfort during the outage, reinforcing the value of their commitment to emergency preparedness.

Pre-made List

Creating a prepper pantry is a proactive step towards ensuring your family's safety during unexpected crises. However, it can be a daunting endeavor, especially for those new to the world of preparedness. To help beginners take those crucial first steps, we've put together a pre-made shopping list that serves as a solid foundation for your stockpile. This basic list is designed to provide you with essential items to kickstart your prepper pantry. As you grow more experienced, you can tailor your stockpile to your family's specific needs and preferences.

Let's delve into this list in more detail:

Canned Goods

Variety of Vegetables: Choose an assortment of canned vegetables like peas, corn, carrots, and green beans. They provide crucial vitamins and minerals for a well-balanced diet.

Fruits: Opt for canned fruits such as peaches, pears, and pineapple. These can be a source of vitamin C and natural sweetness.

Meats: Canned meats like chicken, turkey, and ham are excellent sources of protein and can be used in various recipes.

Soups: Include canned soups with meat and vegetables for satisfying, ready-to-eat meals.

Non-Perishable Staples

Rice: White and brown rice are versatile staples that can be used in a multitude of dishes.
Pasta: Spaghetti, macaroni, and other pasta shapes are filling and easy to store.
Flour: All-purpose flour can be used for baking and cooking.
Sugar: A basic sweetener for beverages and recipes.
Dried Beans: Stock up on varieties like black beans, kidney beans, and lentils, which are rich in protein and fiber.

Dried Grains and Legumes

Quinoa: This gluten-free grain is packed with protein and essential amino acids.
Oats: Oats provide fiber and can be used for breakfast or baking.
Lentils: An excellent source of plant-based protein.

Long-Term Storage Items

Dehydrated Fruits and Vegetables: These have a long shelf life and offer a nutritious snack option.
Freeze-Dried Meals: Perfect for quick, hot meals during emergencies.

Canned or Dried Dairy

Evaporated Milk: A versatile milk option for cooking and drinking.
Powdered Milk: Provides essential calcium and nutrients.
Cheese: Canned or dried cheese adds flavor to various dishes.

Nut Butter

Peanut or Almond Butter: These are excellent sources of protein and healthy fats.

Canned Fish

Tuna, Salmon, or Sardines: Rich in omega-3 fatty acids and protein.

Dried Fruits and Nuts

Raisins, Apricots, Almonds, and Walnuts: These provide essential vitamins, minerals, and healthy fats.

Multivitamins

To supplement essential nutrients and address potential dietary gaps.

Water

A reliable supply of water is crucial for your family's survival. Store an adequate amount, and consider a water purification method as well. We will dive into the depths of this topic later.

This pre-made shopping list provides a diverse range of foods to cater to your family's nutritional needs during emergencies. As you continue building your prepper pantry, remember to rotate items regularly to maintain freshness and avoid waste. Over time, you can expand your stockpile, incorporating your family's dietary preferences and special requirements to ensure their safety and well-being in times of uncertainty.

In the pages that follow, we'll explore how to efficiently organize your prepper pantry and creatively find space in your home for extra food, water, and gear for emergencies. By following these strategies and learning from the success of families like the Peterson's, you'll be well on your way to creating a robust 90-day survival food stockpile, ensuring your family's safety and well-being during a catastrophe.

3

STOCKPILING TECHNIQUES AND PERSONALIZED PREPAREDNESS: STRATEGIES TO SAFEGUARD YOUR FAMILY

"Take care to get what you like or you will be forced to like what you get."

— GEORGE BERNARD SHAW

THE RESILIENCE OF A WELL-PLANNED FOOD SUPPLY

During the most challenging moments of unexpected emergencies, a well-planned food supply can be a lifeline, sustaining your family through adversity. We often underestimate the importance of stockpiling until we hear the stories of those who found themselves unprepared.

Consider the tale of Sarah and John, a couple residing on the outskirts of a small town, who weathered a severe winter storm that left them isolated for weeks. They had lost power and the snow was so deep they could hardly open their front door. However, thanks to their stockpile of food and essentials not only did that ensure their survival, but also inspired them to become advocates for emergency preparedness. Their story underscores the significance of a meticulously planned prepper pantry.

Long-Term Storage: Safeguarding Your Stockpile

Ensuring the long-term viability of your prepper pantry is essential for emergency preparedness. A report by the USDA states that 12.9% of American households were food-insecure at some point during 2021, emphasizing the importance of food storage. Long-term storage practices will not only extend the shelf life of your supplies but also guarantee that your stockpile remains a dependable resource during an unforeseen crises like Sarah and John faced. Here, we will delve into the key principles and strategies of long-term storage.

Optimal Conditions: Protecting Your Investment

The longevity of your stored goods depends significantly on the conditions in which they are stored. Expert tip, here is a fantastic acronym to remember, I know how much prepper's love acronyms! "HALT" stands for the 4 major enemies of shelf-life: humidity, air, light, and temperature. For optimal results, adhere to these essential conditions:

Cool Temperatures: The ideal storage temperature for your prepper pantry is in the range of 50-70 degrees Fahrenheit (10-21 degrees Celsius). This moderate range prevents food from degrading or spoiling prematurely. Extremes of heat can accelerate spoilage, while freezing temperatures may damage the texture and quality of certain items.

Darkness: Sunlight and prolonged exposure to artificial light can degrade the quality of stored food. When possible, store your supplies in a dark area or use opaque containers to shield them from light exposure.

Dry Environment: Moisture is the arch-nemesis of long-term food storage. It can lead to mold, bacterial growth, and the degradation of food quality. To counteract moisture, maintain a dry environment. Basements, crawl spaces, and damp areas should be avoided. Consider using moisture-absorbing products like desiccants to mitigate humidity.

Airtight Containers: Investing in airtight containers or vacuum-sealed bags is a prudent choice. These barriers not only preserve the freshness of your items but also shield them from pests. Insects and rodents can wreak havoc on your supplies, rendering them inedible. Airtight seals keep out air, which contains oxygen that can lead to oxidation and rancidity, further extending the shelf life of your goods.

Oxygen Absorbers: Consider employing various oxygen absorbers in your storage containers. These small packets contain iron powder that reacts with oxygen, reducing the oxygen levels within the container. By minimizing oxygen exposure, you help preserve the nutritional content of your stored food, preventing oxidation and nutrient breakdown over time. This is particularly crucial for items sensitive to oxygen, such as fats and vitamins, ensuring that your emergency stockpile remains a reliable source of essential nutrients for an extended period.

Rotation: Even with the best storage conditions, the inevitable march of time affects all stored food. To counteract this, embrace a strategy of rotation. This practice entails using older items from your stockpile and replenishing them with newer purchases. This ensures that nothing goes to waste and that you always have a fresh supply of goods.

Packaging Considerations

When it comes to long-term storage, the packaging of your supplies plays a pivotal role. Food waste in the United States accounts for 30-40% of the food supply, underlining the importance of efficient pantry management. Take into account these considerations:

Mylar Bags: Mylar bags are excellent for preserving dried goods, like beans, rice, and dehydrated fruits. They provide a reliable barrier against moisture and pests. When used in combination with oxygen absorbers, they create a near-impenetrable storage solution.

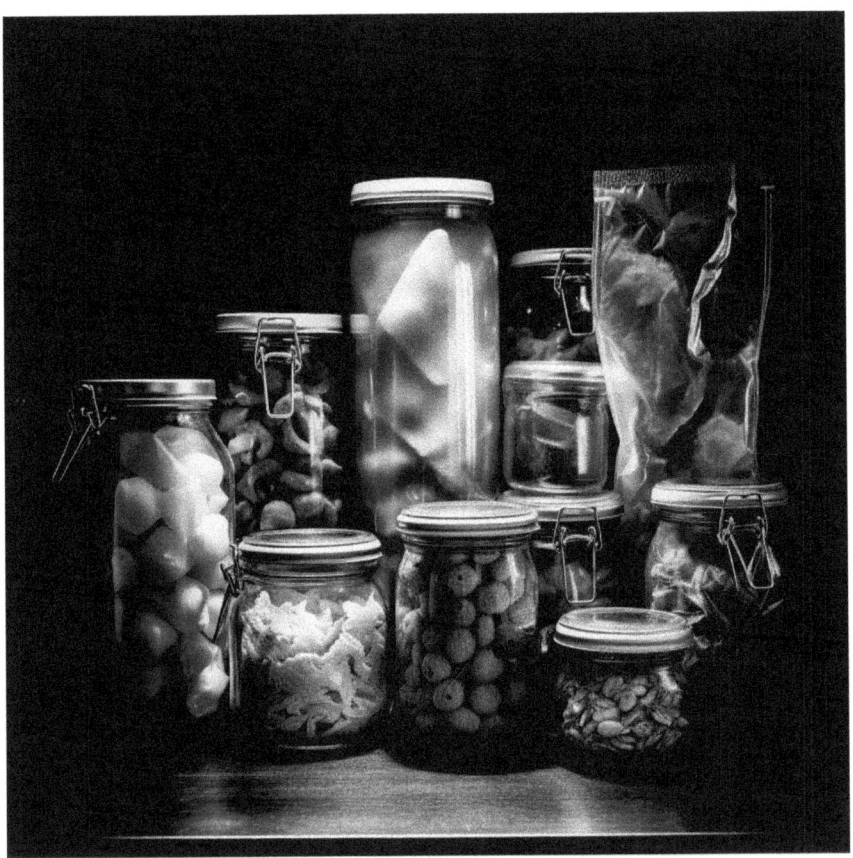

Food-Grade Buckets: Large, food-grade buckets are suitable for storing bulk quantities of grains, legumes, and staples. When coupled with gasket-sealed lids, they create a secure environment for long-term storage.

Glass Jars: Glass jars are particularly useful for preserving dehydrated fruits, nuts, and dried herbs. Their transparent nature allows for quick inspection, and airtight lids keep moisture and air at bay.

Pouches and Foil Packets: Many freeze-dried and dehydrated meals come in individual pouches or foil packets. These are lightweight, convenient, and typically have an extended shelf life. They are perfect for bug-out bags and portable kits.

By observing these long-term storage principles and investing in appropriate containers, you can maintain the quality of your stockpile, prevent waste, and ensure that your family's nutritional needs are met during emergencies. Your prepper pantry will stand as a bastion of preparedness and resilience when it is time to rely on it most.

STOCKPILING AND PREPPING IN SMALL SPACES: OVERCOMING URBAN CHALLENGES

Stockpiling isn't exclusive to spacious homes with ample storage. It's a practice that can be tailored to suit any living space, no matter how modest. Understanding storage considerations and infrastructure is key to maximizing the efficiency of your prepper pantry. Living in an urban environment, such as an apartment, can present unique challenges for stockpiling and prepping. Space constraints, building regulations, and the transient nature of urban life can all complicate your preparedness efforts. However, with careful planning and strategic thinking, it's entirely possible to create a well-stocked and resilient prepper pantry within these limitations. Let's explore some vital considerations.

Storage Space Options in Small Spaces

Space is the most obvious challenge in urban areas, where every square foot is precious. In smaller living quarters, creativity becomes your ally. A study by the Red Cross found that 53% of Americans have less than three days' worth of non-perishable food at home. If you live in the city, do not make that your excuse to not have at least a few week's of food and supplies stored up for a worst-case scenario event. To maximize your storage capacity for space and stockpile, consider the following strategies:

Under-Bed Storage: Utilize the space under your bed for storage bins. These can hold non-perishable items, water containers, or supplies.

Wall-Mounted Shelving: Install sturdy wall shelves to take advantage of vertical space. Use these shelves for items that aren't too heavy, like canned goods and essential supplies.

Closet Shelving: Install additional shelving in your closets to create pantry space. Clear, stackable containers will keep items organized and visible.

Furniture with Storage: Invest in multi-functional furniture with hidden storage compartments. Ottomans, coffee tables, and beds with built-in drawers can all provide extra space.

Over-Door Organizers: Hang over-door organizers on the inside of pantry doors to store smaller items like spices, condiments, and hygiene products.

ESSENTIALS FOR SMALL SPACE STOCKPILING

In small spaces, it's crucial to prioritize the most essential items while making the best use of available room. Do not let apartment living be the reason you do not have extra food and supplies! Key items to include:

Non-Perishable Foods: Opt for canned goods, dehydrated or freeze-dried foods, pasta, rice, and other staples with long shelf lives.

Water Storage: Space-saving water containers, like stackable water bricks or collapsible water containers, can help store an adequate water supply.

Hygiene Products: Stick to compact sizes of soap, shampoo, and other hygiene products. Look for concentrated or multi-purpose items to save space.

Medical Supplies: Focus on first-aid essentials, prescription medications, and basic medical tools like thermometers and bandages.

Cooking Gear: Choose versatile cooking equipment that doesn't take up too much space. Portable stoves, lightweight cookware, and utensils are ideal.

Alternative Energy Sources: Consider compact solar chargers for small electronic devices and LED lanterns for lighting.

BUILDING REGULATIONS AND LEASES

Urban living often means dealing with building regulations and rental agreements. Before making significant changes to your apartment for stockpiling, review your lease or building regulations. Ensure you're compliant with any rules regarding shelving, modifications, and types of items you can store.

Transience and Mobility

Urban areas tend to have a more transient population. People move frequently, so your stockpile should be portable and easy to disassemble. Opt for lightweight and stackable storage containers that you can easily pack up if you move to a new apartment.

Community and Cooperation

In urban settings, community resources and cooperation can be invaluable. Consider joining local prepper groups or neighborhood associations to pool resources and knowledge. Sharing a bulk purchase of items, like rice or canned goods, with neighbors can save space and money.

Urban Preparedness is Possible

Prepping in an urban environment is challenging, but not impossible. With creative storage solutions, smart choices in what to stockpile, and a flexible mindset, you can create a reliable prepper pantry even in a small apartment. Urban preparedness is all about making the most of limited resources and building a sense of community resilience. By investing time and effort into your small space stockpile, you'll be better prepared for whatever challenges come your way in the city.

OPTIMIZING SPACE IN LARGER HOMES

In more spacious homes, optimizing space is equally important. Large pantries, second pantries, or basement storage can quickly become disorganized if not structured efficiently. Here are some additional strategies to make the most of your available space:

Shelving Units: Installing shelving units can be a game-changer. Consider adjustable shelving that can be customized to fit different-sized items. Additionally, wire shelving allows for proper ventilation, preventing moisture buildup.

Clear Containers: Invest in clear, airtight containers for food storage. These not only keep your stockpile organized but also protect items from pests and moisture while keeping them visible.

Label Everything: Labeling your containers and shelves can save you time and help keep your pantry organized. It's easier to find what you need when items are clearly marked.

Rolling Storage: Consider rolling storage solutions for larger items like water barrels and heavy supplies. These can be moved easily, allowing you to access items at the back of the storage area without hassle.

Temperature Control: In larger homes, temperature fluctuations can impact food storage. Consider adding a thermometer to your pantry to monitor temperature changes. Installing insulation or climate control solutions can also help.

Rotation System: Implement a rotation system for your stockpile. This involves using older items first to ensure nothing expires or goes to waste. Regularly check and update your inventory to maintain freshness.

Emergency Planning Zone: Dedicate a specific area in your larger home to serve as an emergency planning zone. This is where you can keep your emergency kits, medical supplies, and important documents, ensuring easy access during a crisis.

By incorporating these strategies into your larger home, you'll make the most of your space while ensuring your prepper pantry remains well-organized, accessible, and ready for any emergency.

WATER AND OTHER ESSENTIAL SUPPLIES

Water, the elixir of life, stands as the crown jewel of your stockpile. Adequate supplies of water and essential items form the backbone of your emergency preparedness. It's not just about having enough food; it's about addressing all aspects of survival. Water is #1 on this list, so important that I wrote an entire book just on this topic titled Water for Survival: Essential Techniques, Tools, and Tips to Survive Any Water Emergency. Although not as in-depth as my book, here's a water section discussing why it will be part of your family's stockpile:

Water

Your top priority, water is vital for hydration, cooking, hygiene, and growing crops as necessary. Adequate supplies should cover drinking, sanitation, and medical needs. Experts recommend storing at least one gallon of water per person per day. Expert tip, where there is space double that total. Water purification methods, like filters and chemical treatments, should also be part of your stockpile for extended emergencies. The best aspect of these is they can become portable, and they take up very little space. We have a Potable Aqua or iodine tablets in every BOB. In a national survey, 64% of respondents said they have experienced food or water shortages during a disaster so don't let that be you!

Here's a more detailed exploration of water storage considerations for your prepper pantry:

Water Quantity and Duration: The first consideration is how much water you need and for how long. FEMA recommends storing at least one gallon of water per person per day for at least three days. However, during extended emergencies or natural disasters, you may need more. Aim for a two-week supply as a minimum, but if possible, strive for a 30-day supply. Since this is the Ultimate Prepper Pantry Guide I would make a goal of 90-days worth for the family. Expert tip, if you are on a well, obtain a hand pump for your well. Some styles of hand pumps can be mounted on a well without disrupting your existing electric well pump, and be used as a backup to deal with power outages. Another part of our water emergency plan is to take 5 gallon buckets with lids to our creek in the back and run that water through our Crown Berkey in our home. Keep in mind that water is not just for drinking; it's also necessary for hygiene and food preparation. Sourcing rainwater is another great option for non-drinking water needs. I go into much depth in my Water for Survival book on this topic.

Water Storage Containers: The quality and suitability of your water storage containers are critical. Choose food-grade containers designed for long-term water storage. These can include water jugs, barrels, or stackable water bricks. Ensure they have tight-fitting, screw-on lids to prevent contamination.

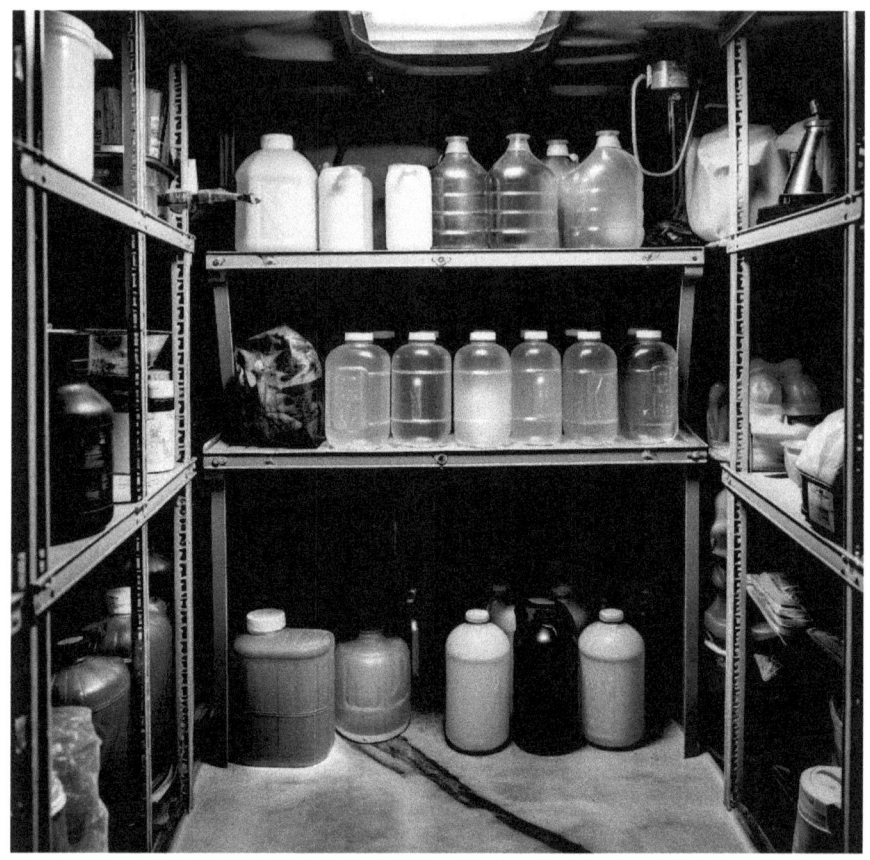

Water Treatment: Over time, stored water can become stagnant and potentially develop bacteria or algae. To combat this, consider using water preservers or chlorine bleach (unscented) to treat your stored water. Follow recommended guidelines for water treatment and use proper storage rotation to maintain water quality.

Location: Store your water containers in a cool, dark, and dry location. Avoid exposing them to direct sunlight or extreme temperature fluctuations, as this can compromise the containers over time. Basements or dark closets are suitable places.

Filtration and Purification: In case your stored water runs out, or if you need to source water from natural sources, it's wise to have water filtration and purification methods on hand. Portable water filters and purification tablets can make contaminated water safe to drink. These are crucial for long-term sustainability.

Hygiene Water: In addition to drinking water, you'll need water for hygiene purposes, such as handwashing, bathing, and cleaning. Consider the use of a separate water source, like a hand-pumped well or rainwater harvesting system, for non-potable water needs.

Storage Rotation: To ensure the freshness of your stored water, practice a regular rotation schedule. This involves using the older water and replacing it with fresh supplies. A first-in, first-out (FIFO) system is a simple way to manage this.

Water Monitoring: Periodically check your water containers for any signs of damage, leaks, or contamination. Regular maintenance and monitoring ensure your water supply remains reliable.

Rainwater Harvesting: If possible, consider setting up a rainwater harvesting system. This allows you to collect and store rainwater, reducing your reliance on pre-purchased water. Ensure the system is legal in your area and follows all safety guidelines.

Backup Water Sources: In the event your stored water supply runs out, it's essential to have backup sources. Identify nearby natural water sources like rivers, lakes, or ponds that can be accessed if needed. Ensure you have the necessary filtration and purification methods to make this water safe to consume.

By paying close attention to water storage considerations and actively managing your water supply, you can ensure that your family has access to clean, safe water during emergencies, helping to safeguard their health and well-being.

Hygiene Products

Maintaining personal hygiene is crucial during emergencies to prevent illness. Stockpile items like soap, hand sanitizer, toothpaste, toilet paper, feminine hygiene products, and diapers for infants. A portable camp shower may also prove invaluable for bathing when regular water sources are unavailable.

Medical Supplies

A comprehensive first-aid kit should include bandages, antiseptics, pain relievers, prescription medications, and any necessary medical equipment for family members with chronic conditions. Additionally, consider stockpiling items like thermometers, blood pressure cuffs, and basic diagnostic tools.

COOKING UTENSILS AND POWERLESS KITCHEN SUPPLIES

In the event of power outages or restricted resources, having alternative kitchen supplies is essential, and often overlooked. Here is a short list of powerless utensils often overlooked that should be in your stockpile supplies:

Manual Can Opener: In a world where electric can openers are the norm, a manual can opener is a prepper's best friend. Ensure you have a sturdy and reliable one in your pantry to access canned goods without the need for electricity.

Hand-Cranked Appliances: Hand-cranked appliances like hand mixers, blenders, and coffee grinders can provide a means of food preparation without electricity. Look for durable options with good reviews.

Manual Coffee Maker: For coffee lovers, a manual coffee maker like a French press or a pour-over system is a must. It allows you to brew your morning coffee without electricity.

Manual Food Processor: A manual food processor can chop, slice, and dice your ingredients without the need for a power source. It's a versatile tool for meal preparation.

Manual Grain Mill: If you store whole grains for flour, a manual grain mill can help you turn them into usable flour for baking. It's a handy tool for making bread or other grain-based dishes.

Mortar and Pestle: This ancient tool is perfect for grinding spices, herbs, and small amounts of grains or seeds. It's ideal for flavoring your meals without relying on electric grinders.

Manual Egg Beater: Whipping up eggs or batters with a manual egg beater is both efficient and fun. It's a simple but effective tool for your kitchen.

Hand-Cranked Radio: While not a kitchen utensil, a hand-cranked radio can keep you informed during emergencies. Many hand-cranked radios also come with built-in flashlights and USB plug-ins for charging phones, tablets, lanterns, headlamps for added utility.

Hand-Operated Water Pump: If you have water stored in large containers, a hand-operated water pump makes it easy to access the water without lifting heavy containers.

Manual Ice Cream Maker: Ice cream might seem like a luxury during a crisis, but it can boost morale. A manual ice cream maker allows you to enjoy this treat even without electricity.

Mechanical Kitchen Timer: Accurate timing is crucial for cooking and baking. A mechanical kitchen timer is a reliable tool that doesn't rely on batteries.

Manual Juicer: Freshly squeezed juice can provide essential vitamins during emergencies. A manual juicer can extract juice from fruits without electricity.

Hand-Crank Flashlight: While not a kitchen tool, a hand-crank flashlight can be kept in your pantry to ensure you have a reliable source of light during power outages. These do not require batteries, hence the hand-crank part, and are also awesome items for each bug out bag.

By including these motorless kitchen utensils and tools in your prepper pantry, you'll be better equipped to prepare meals, stay informed, and maintain a sense of normalcy during emergencies, regardless of power availability.

BACK-UP POWER SOURCES AND ALTERNATIVE COOKING METHODS

When disaster strikes, power outages can be common, and having a reliable source of electricity and alternative methods for cooking becomes crucial. In this section, we'll delve deeper into these aspects of prepping:

Back-Up Power Sources

Generators: Portable generators can provide temporary power during outages. They come in various sizes and power capacities, so choose one that suits your needs. Remember to store fuel safely, and regularly maintain the generator to ensure it functions when needed.This is a topic

I will not touch as I know every prepper has their strong opinion on capacity, type, brand, and style. Use common sense to get what fits your family's needs in the home you are in.

Solar Power: Solar panels and power banks are an eco-friendly way to generate electricity. They're an excellent long-term solution but may have a higher upfront cost. Look for portable solar chargers to keep essential devices like phones and lights running.

Battery Banks: Battery banks, such as lithium-ion power stations, store electrical energy for later use. They can charge phones, power lights, and even small appliances. Consider their capacity, ease of use, and recharge options.

Car Power Inverters: These devices allow you to convert your car's battery power into AC electricity. They're handy for charging smaller devices or running low-power appliances during short-term power outages.

Hand-Cranked Devices: As discussed, hand-cranked radios, flashlights, and phone chargers can provide essential power during emergencies. They are a great value and again, don't require batteries or an external power source, making them ideal for off-grid situations.

ALTERNATIVE COOKING METHODS

As reliable as propane, gas, or electric can be to fuel your home, if you are in a major emergency type event, odds are good you may not be able to access this energy for some duration of time. How do you stay warm or cook food? Here are a few alternative options for your stockpile that are versatile enough to use while camping too.

Camp Stoves: Portable camp stoves are an excellent backup for cooking during power outages. They run on propane or butane and are relatively easy to use. Ensure you have a sufficient supply of fuel canisters.

Wood-Burning Stoves: If you have access to firewood, a wood-burning stove can be a reliable alternative for cooking and heating. They come in various designs, from traditional to more modern, efficient models.

Charcoal Grills: Charcoal grills can function as a makeshift oven. With a little practice, you can use them to bake, roast, or even cook stovetop dishes. They're handy for short-term power outages.

Solar Ovens: Solar ovens use sunlight to cook food. They are eco-friendly and suitable for long-term power disruptions. However, they require ample sunlight and may take longer to prepare meals.

Camping Cookware: Have a set of camping cookware on hand, including pots, pans, and utensils. They are designed for use over open flames or portable stoves and can be used for alternative cooking.

Fire Pit or Grill: If you have outdoor space, a fire pit or grill can be used for open-fire cooking. It's essential to know local regulations and safety guidelines when using open flames.

Having reliable back-up power sources and alternative cooking methods in your prepper pantry ensures that you can maintain essential functions, like lighting, warmth, communication, and meal preparation, even during extended power outages. Choose options that align with your needs, space, and environmental considerations. Regularly test and maintain these devices to keep them in working order, providing peace of mind in the face of unexpected emergencies.

STOCKPILING DIFFERENT FAMILY SIZES

Stockpiling is not a one-size-fits-all endeavor. Every family has unique needs based on its composition and demographics. From single individuals to extended families and even our beloved pets, each group requires tailored strategies for stockpiling. As the demographics of families evolve, it's essential to adapt your emergency preparedness accordingly. In the United States, extended and blended families are on the rise, emphasizing the need for flexibility in stockpiling strategies.

Let's explore how to meet the needs of various family sizes:

Single Individuals: Singles can stockpile effectively, focusing on compact and versatile items. It's also a chance to build a community of prepared friends or neighbors who can provide support during a crisis.

Elderly Couples: Consider health and dietary restrictions while stockpiling. Ensure that medical necessities, prescription medications, and mobility aids are available. If mobility is an issue, have a plan for assistance or evacuation in place.

Married Couples: Stockpile based on dietary preferences, lifestyle, and any health conditions. Engage both partners in the process to ensure a well-rounded pantry. Having clearly defined roles and responsibilities can streamline the process and ease decision-making.

Extended Families: With the rise of extended and blended families, coordination is key. Ensure that stockpile items cater to the diverse needs and preferences of family members. Discuss and delegate responsibilities to avoid duplication and ensure that everyone's needs are met.

Infants and Young Children: Stockpile baby food, formula, diapers, and hygiene products. Ensure that medical items and specialized care are readily available. Additionally, consider entertainment and comfort items to keep children calm during emergencies. The American Academy of Pediatrics recommends that families have at least a two-week supply of food and water in their emergency preparedness kits to ensure children's well-being during disasters. This can be overlooked with small children when doing stockpile calculation needs.

Pets: Don't forget your furry companions. Stock up on pet food, medications, and any necessary pet care items to ensure their well-being during crises. Plan for the emotional support and security pets offer.

As the landscape of families in the United States evolves, so should our emergency preparedness strategies. Whether you're stocking up for one or for many, the ultimate goal remains the same: ensuring the safety and well-being of your loved ones in the face of adversity.

In times of crisis, the choices you make today will determine your family's comfort, security, and survival. The careful selection and storage of essential supplies, from food and water to power sources and cooking methods, form the backbone of your preparedness. This chapter has equipped you with the knowledge to navigate these critical considerations effectively.

Remember that preparedness is not a one-size-fits-all endeavor. Each family is unique, with varying needs and circumstances. Whether you're stockpiling for a single person, a growing family, or even pets, the principles of preparedness remain the same: thoughtful planning, strategic organization, and adaptable strategies.

Your prepper pantry is more than just a physical space filled with supplies. It represents your commitment to the safety, comfort, and well-being of your loved ones, even in the face of adversity. By applying the techniques and strategies outlined in this chapter, you are taking proactive steps toward ensuring that your family is prepared for the unknown.

4

DISCOVER MEAL PLANNING BASICS FROM YOUR FOOD STOCKPILE: CRAFTING HARMONY THROUGH 90 DAYS OF FLOURISHING PANTRY PROVISIONS

"Stockpiling food is a form of self-reliance and self-respect."

— MEL TAPPAN

THRIVING THROUGH ADVERSITY

When disaster struck unexpectedly, the Ortiz family found themselves relying on an advanced 90-day meal plan they meticulously crafted for their survival pantry. Months earlier, they had researched, calculated, and carefully organized their prepper pantry, considering every detail from family preferences to nutritional needs. As shelves emptied and grocery stores became inaccessible, their comprehensive meal plan emerged as a beacon of stability for a few months. From creative breakfast oats, to versatile canned meal combinations for lunch, and comforting dinners crafted from pantry staples, each meal brought not just sustenance but a sense of normalcy. The Ortiz's navigated adversity with resilience, thanks to their proactive meal planning—a testament to foresight and preparation in the face of unexpected challenges.

In uncertain times, meeting your family's nutrition and emotional needs is crucial. This chapter dives into the essential world of stockpile meal planning, and general stockpile inventory management, guiding you not just to survive but thrive for 90 days from your pantry. Understanding diverse meals, nutritional balance, and smart planning helps you face challenges with strength. Plus, mixing in creative meals and rotating them keeps things adaptable during uncertainty. In the midst of adversity, nutrition is the cornerstone of resilience. Advanced meal planning to suit your specific family needs will create a seamless flow within your food stockpile and prepper journey.

MEAL PLANNING FOR 90 DAYS OF SURVIVAL

Planning Your Meals

First and foremost, it's essential to figure out what you and your family enjoy eating. So have a family meeting with the goal to come away with 20 meals written down that you all enjoy. Another option is to simply pay attention at meal time over the next month and record the feedback as your data points. In our house we have about 30 go-to meals that my wife has recorded that all 6 of us will enjoy eating. Starting with food you all enjoy is the foundation for crafting a meal plan that not only sustains you but also brings comfort and familiarity during trying times. Segmenting meals into breakfast, lunch, dinner, and complementary sides is not just about delineating eating times; it's about creating a holistic nutritional plan. Let's breakdown mealtime options.

Breakfast

Breakfast stands as the cornerstone of a well-rounded day, especially during uncertain times. It kick-starts metabolism and fuels the body and mind. When planning meals using your prepper pantry, ensuring a hearty and nutritious breakfast becomes paramount. Stocking essentials like oats, dried fruits, nuts, and powdered milk facilitates crafting wholesome breakfast options. Incorporating long-lasting items such as whole-grain cereals or canned fruits ensures a reliable morning meal that sustains energy levels through the day's challenges. If you're lucky enough to have chickens, then your egg source is secured as well! If there are no chickens, there will already be a stocked pantry if you follow my plan.

For breakfast, it's a good idea to have a variety of options. Choose 10 different breakfast meals and multiply them by

40 to create a plan that's a little more than a year's worth. While this may seem like a lot, the goal is to make the math as straightforward as possible.

10 Breakfast Meals x 40 = 400 Breakfast Meals for the Year

Lunch

Lunch offers a much-needed pause, refueling energy and focus for the rest of the day. Utilizing your prepper pantry for mid-day meals involves thoughtful planning. Canned proteins like tuna or beans, combined with shelf-stable grains and vegetables, allow for versatile and satisfying lunches. Incorporating items like canned soups or dehydrated vegetables facilitates quick and nourishing meal preparations, ensuring a balanced mid-day break that supports sustained productivity.

In a survival scenario, preparing three large hot meals daily may not be practical. You'll be fortunate to manage one. For lunch, consider having enough ingredients to make bread at least once a day. Bread can be used for various purposes, including making sandwiches, rolls with leftover meat, toast, and more.

1 loaf of Bread x 365 = 365 Loafs of Bread

Dinner

Dinner holds a special place as a time for family bonding and unwinding. Leveraging your prepper pantry for dinner staples involves considering comforting and versatile ingredients. Items like canned tomatoes, pasta, rice, or beans become versatile bases for hearty dinners. Incorporating shelf-stable sauces, spices, and condiments ensures flavor diversity. Planning for dinners with your prepper pantry involves creating meals that not only provide nourishment, but also foster a sense of togetherness and normalcy during challenging times. Dinner, typically your main meal of the day, should be thoughtfully organized. Categorize your meals into four groups: Soup, Salad, & Appetizer Meals; Beans & Mexican Meals; Rice & Chicken Meals; and Pasta & Italian Meals. With nine different meals in each category, you'll have a variety of options to choose from.

9 Meals of Each Category x 4 = 36 Different Dinners
36 Dinners x 10 = 360 Dinners

To maintain a well-rotated food stockpile, aim to prepare at least two meals from your food storage each week. Most of the ingredients you store should have a minimum 3-year shelf-life, and by rotating your food this way, you can help ensure that nothing goes to waste.

Side Dishes

Side dishes add depth and completeness to meals, complementing the main course with flavors and textures. When leveraging your prepper pantry for side dishes, it's about maximizing simplicity without compromising taste. Canned vegetables, such as green beans or corn, offer convenience and nutritional value. Shelf-stable grains like quinoa or couscous can serve as versatile bases for side salads or pilafs. Additionally, dehydrated herbs or seasoning blends elevate flavors without the need for fresh ingredients. Incorporating these pantry items into side dishes not only adds variety but also contributes essential nutrients, making meals more satisfying and well-rounded. It will depend on your family, but we do not need a side for every meal (especially if we are rationing in an emergency). Of the four groups section up above, you could likely get away with meal planning using sides in 2 of these categories.

9 sides of x 2 of selected Categories (not all 4) = 18 Different Meals (sides can be used with lunch or dinner)
18 Sides x 10 = 180 Sides

Dessert

Let's not forget dessert! Add about 3 desserts a week to your plan. Comfort foods and snacks are essential in your food storage. After all, desserts can count as a meal, right?

15 Desserts x 10 = 150 Desserts

For those who lean toward a diet centered around fruits and vegetables, there are still ways to incorporate food storage into your meal planning. I have discussed each of these options more in-depth in other sections of our ultimate prepper pantry survival guide, but they can be touched on again here together for planning meal purposes for the vegetarians in your group.

Learn to Cook the Staples: Even if you don't consume wheat, beans, or other staples daily, consider learning to cook with them. These foods have exceptionally long shelf lives and can be a valuable addition to your food storage for times of need.

Freeze-dry: Freeze-dried foods retain most of their original nutritional value and have a shelf life of over 25 years. Consider sampling some small pantry cans to experience the convenience and versatility they offer.

Can it: Canning your favorite fruits and vegetables is an excellent way to enhance your food storage. It allows you to plan for sides like green beans, peaches, or other favorites, even when fresh produce is not available.

Start a Garden: As we will discuss in length, a garden can be a valuable addition to your prepper toolkit. Whether it's a few containers and sprouts or a complete backyard transformation, gardening skills are essential if you want to maintain a diet rich in fresh produce. You can also invest in a can of seeds, which can remain viable for over 20 years in the freezer.

By harnessing strategic organization, culinary diversity, and resourceful utilization, meal planning becomes a conduit for stability, providing sustenance and comfort when it's needed most. Remember, this journey toward culinary preparedness is not solely about food—it's about safeguarding a sense of normalcy and security for you and your loved ones amidst adversity.

INVENTORY MANAGEMENT TOOLS FOR AN ORGANIZED PANTRY

Accurate record-keeping is crucial for effective pantry management. Keeping track of what you buy and store ensures you stay organized and reduce waste. There are various tools available to help you manage your prepper pantry inventory:

Pantry Organization Online Spreadsheet

Creating your own inventory spreadsheet allows for customization based on your needs. You can create a food stockpile spreadsheet using online tools like Excel or Google Sheets. These platforms allow you to organize your meals, quantities, and dates efficiently. If you prefer a ready-made one, look for the free gift link to download mine! This is a practical tool that you can use as a template for your food stockpile inventory list, this is not intended as a meal planner. It's designed to streamline your record-keeping and assist you in keeping your pantry organized, efficient, and up-to-date.

Here are some tips on spreadsheet headers and vital information to track:

Item Name: Clearly label each item in your stockpile. Use a consistent and descriptive name to avoid confusion.

Category: Group items into categories, such as canned goods, grains, pasta, spices, and condiments. This makes it easier to locate specific items when needed.

Quantity: Keep track of the quantity of each item in your stockpile. This helps you know when you're running low and need to restock. Unit of measure may be needed in a separate column depending on how you organize it.

Purchase Date: Record the date when you acquired each item. This is crucial for FIFO (First In, First Out) rotation and helps you use older items before newer ones.

Expiration Date: Include the expiration date, best-by date, or use-by date for each item. This information is vital for managing the freshness and safety of your stockpile.

Storage Location: Note where each item is stored in your pantry, basement, or bulk storage area. This helps you quickly locate items when needed.

Notes: Use this section for additional information, such as special storage requirements, important details about the item, or notes about past usage or preferences.

MEAL PLANNING ONLINE SPREADSHEET

There are countless numbers of online boot camps, courses, books, and websites specializing in meal planning strategies. Declaring a singular "best" plan is challenging due to the multitude of factors—family size, dietary needs, preferences, environmental conditions, and geographical locations—each influencing meal planning differently. What I can share is what has proven effective for us when putting together a meal planning strategy for the apocalypse. It serves as a reliable starting point for many families, providing a solid baseline to begin their meal planning journey.

Categorize your meals into breakfast, lunch, and dinner for easy reference. Include details such as ingredients, preparation instructions, and links to recipes if needed.

Breakfast Column:

Row Entries: List specific breakfast options (oatmeal, dry cereal, etc.).
Ingredients Column: Detail necessary ingredients for each breakfast option.
Preparation Instructions Column: Include step-by-step directions for preparing each breakfast meal.

Lunch Column:

Row Entries: Specify lunch options (bean salads, canned soups, sandwiches, etc.).

Ingredients Column: Enumerate required ingredients for each lunch choice.

Preparation Instructions Column: Provide instructions on how to assemble or prepare each lunch item.

Dinner Column:

Row Entries: List dinner meal choices (pasta dishes, rice and beans, etc.).

Ingredients Column: Outline ingredients needed for each dinner recipe.

Preparation Instructions Column: Offer detailed steps to cook or assemble each dinner option.

Spreadsheet Organization Tips:

Color Coding: Use different colors for breakfast, lunch, and dinner sections for quick identification.

Hyperlinks: Embed links to online recipes or instructions for complex meals.

Portion Sizes: Consider adding columns for portion sizes or serving suggestions for better planning.

Use the spreadsheet to track your meal plan for the entire month. It's a digital reference that ensures you never have to wonder what's for dinner. By organizing your meal plan into categories with detailed ingredient lists and preparation instructions within a spreadsheet, it becomes a user-friendly reference guide, ensuring efficient and varied meal preparation from your prepper pantry supplies.

A Magnetic Board as a Backup

While an online spreadsheet is a fantastic tool, it's crucial to remember that during emergencies or extended power outages, digital resources may not be accessible. In such cases, a magnetic board and magnetic paper can be a valuable backup option. (A white board with dry erase markers is sufficient too) This tangible meal planning board allows you to maintain your meal plan even when the grid goes down. A suggestion would be to create labels for your menu board, based on the meals you've planned. You can also design your labels if you're familiar with graphic design. Print these labels onto magnetic paper, cut them out neatly and put it all together. This is not a "meal planning workshop", simply a starting point for you to get inspired. Please feel free to search online for more in-depth detail on what works for families meal planning and pantry organization needs.

Food Organization Apps: There are several smartphone apps designed to make it easier to manage your inventory. I personally do not use one, but check your app store for one that fits for you. They allow you to input items, quantities, purchase dates, and expiration dates, providing you with alerts for approaching expiration dates. Recipes are preloaded on some pantry apps, and several allow you to manually add recipes for your convenience. These apps are user-friendly and enable you to access your inventory on the go.

Watch Out for Bored Eaters - Rotate Meals!

To keep everyone satisfied and prevent meal fatigue, it's crucial to rotate your meals regularly. This ensures that you and your family don't get bored of the same meals repeating. By cycling through your meal plan, you can provide a diverse and enjoyable dining experience, even during challenging times.

People often wonder if I really eat the food from my storage, and my answer is a resounding "YES!" The key is to store meals that you genuinely enjoy. Food storage isn't just about stockpiling staples like wheat and beans; it's about finding ways to store and efficiently manage the foods you love.

Incorporating this meal planning system into your prepper pantry strategy ensures not only a well-organized approach to food storage, but also peace of mind. With the right plan, you'll have the confidence that you and your family will be well-nourished, even when faced with adversity. Meal planning is not just about food; it's about ensuring that everyone in your family remains content and satisfied, no matter the circumstances.

Your prepper pantry is a testament to your commitment to your family's health and resilience. As you stock it with a thoughtful selection of foods representing essential food groups, you empower your loved ones to face adversity with strength, morale, and a sense of security. If you decide to organize the pantry with a spreadsheet or app, as well as begin creating tasty meals planning for your family in a crisis, this chapter is an excellent starting point for those needs.

Remember that preparedness is a continuous journey. Regularly evaluate and update your stockpile, stay informed about potential risks, and adapt your strategies to evolving circumstances. By investing in your family's nutritional well-being through your prepper pantry, you're not only enhancing their chances of survival but also providing comfort and peace in a world where the unexpected can happen at any moment.

5

PROPER STORAGE MAINTENANCE AND ROTATION OF YOUR FOOD STOCKPILE: EATING WELL TODAY, PREPARING FOR TOMORROW

"The pantry is the heart of the home."

— CARLA HALL

THE FORGOTTEN PROVISIONS

In the midst of a catastrophic flood, Mark and his family had to rely on their well-prepared prepper pantry to sustain them. But as they scoured their stockpile for supplies, they discovered a disheartening reality — some of their food had expired, and their efforts to maintain a functioning food reserve had fallen short. This cautionary tale underscores the critical importance of proper storage maintenance and rotation in your food stockpile.

Implementing an Inventory System

To avoid the disappointment that Mark and his family experienced, it's vital to establish an effective inventory system. In this chapter, we will delve into the significance of our "3-tier food storage method" as the foundation for organized stockpiling.

3-TIER FOOD STORAGE METHOD EXPLAINED (AND RECOMMENDED!)

The 3-tier food storage method is a comprehensive approach to food preparedness, providing a structured and strategic way to ensure a household's nutritional needs during times of emergency or crisis. Each tier has a distinct purpose and goal, with common foods found at each tier. This simple and effective method categorizes your food stockpile into three tiers: Tier 1 (daily pantry), Tier 2 (mid-tier pantry), and Tier 3 (bulk food pantry). It will not only help you manage your supplies efficiently, but also ensures that you consume food before it expires.

Tier 1: The "daily pantry," or tier 1 serves as the foundation of a prepper's food storage strategy. It is intended to provide a 30-60 day supply of food, focusing on the short-term needs of a family. This tier contains items that you and your family consume regularly and can sustain you during initial disruptions. Common foods found in Tier 1 may include canned goods, crackers, sauces, pasta, rice, beans, shelf-stable dairy products, canned fruits and vegetables, and other non-perishable items that have a relatively short shelf life.

Tier 2: The "mid-tier pantry," or tier 2 is designed for mid-term food storage. This tier typically involves creating a basement pantry or storage area with an additional 90 days' supply as the goal. It contains items that have a longer shelf life and are suitable for sustaining your family beyond the initial crisis period. Common foods in Tier 2 might include larger quantities of the items found in Tier 1, as well as items like freeze-dried foods, grains, flour, baking supplies, and more substantial canned goods. This is a great spot to keep larger water containers as well.

Tier 3: the "bulk food pantry," or tier 3 is the long-term food stockpile, intended to sustain your family for an extended period. The goal for Tier 3 is to have foods that can last anywhere from 120 days to 2 years or more. Common foods in Tier 3 are typically freeze-dried or dehydrated foods, grains, legumes, bulk staples like sugar and salt, and various preserved foods in larger quantities. I have vitamins and several water treatment droplets or pills in this section of our bulk food pantry section. We have a back-up ammunition case containing several hundred rounds and a Costco size box of AA and AAA batteries in the tier 3 area. This is not every preppers setup, it just fits with my layout. This tier provides the ultimate level of self-sufficiency, offering a sense of security during prolonged emergencies or disruptions.

In summary, the 3-tier food storage method provides a well-rounded strategy for food preparedness, with each tier serving a specific purpose in terms of supply duration and types of food stored. By diversifying your food storage across these tiers and keeping things organized, you can ensure that your family has access to the necessary nutrition during various stages of an emergency, creating a more comprehensive and sustainable prepping plan.

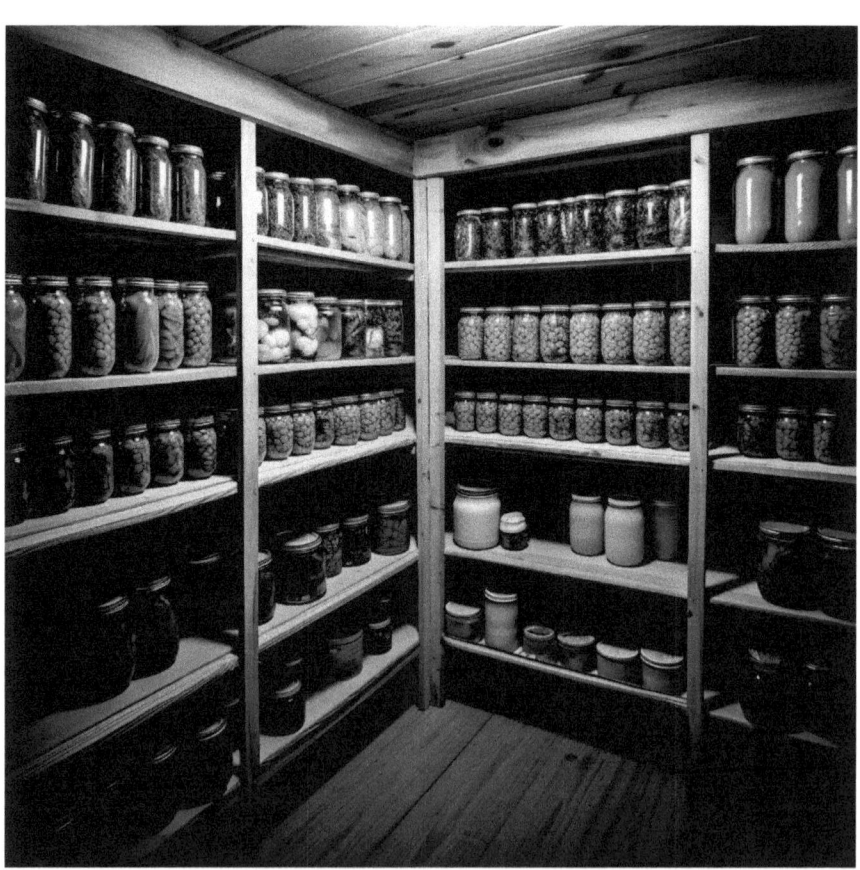

FIFO Method: "First In, First Out" is one of the key strategies for proper rotation. This principle emphasizes consuming the oldest items in your stockpile before the newer ones. By following this simple rule, you ensure that nothing lingers in storage for too long. The benefits are clear: it helps maintain freshness, prevents waste, and allows you to use your stockpile more effectively during emergencies. The first in, first out approach seamlessly integrates with the 3-tier food storage method to form a robust and efficient strategy for building your ultimate food stockpile.

MAINTAINING AN ORGANIZED STORAGE SPACE

A well-organized storage space is essential to ensure that your food stockpile remains in top condition. Here are some detailed tips and strategies for maintaining an organized and efficient storage area:

Easy Access: Store frequently used items in the most accessible areas. Place them at eye level and within arm's reach. This prevents you from having to dig through your stockpile in emergencies.

Efficient Inventory Management: Group similar items together. Create sections for canned goods, dry goods, grains, and other categories, making it easier to locate what you need quickly. Use clear bins or containers to see the contents easily.

Labeling: Label containers with the purchase date and expiration date. This practice helps with the FIFO method and keeps you informed about when to use items. Use a permanent marker or labeling tape for clear, legible labeling.

Appropriate Containers: Choose the right storage containers based on the type of food. I must list a few here to describe which container best fits which environment. You will get your own rhythm of what works best in your home, depending on your pantry size, availability of equipment, your families food preferences, and several other factors.

Airtight Containers for Grains and Dry Goods: Use airtight containers to store grains, flour, sugar, and other dry goods. These containers create a sealed environment that prevents moisture, air, and pests from compromising your food's quality. Look for containers with secure locking mechanisms and rubber gaskets to ensure an airtight seal.

Transparent Containers for Quick Visibility: Consider transparent or semi-transparent containers for items like pasta, rice, and legumes. Being able to see the contents without opening the container simplifies inventory management. It allows you to quickly identify what you have and when it needs replenishing.

Mylar Bags for Long-Term Storage: Mylar bags are excellent for extended storage of bulk items like grains, beans, and dehydrated foods. These bags are designed to protect against light, moisture, and oxygen. When combined with oxygen absorbers, they create a near-perfect storage environment. Be sure to seal them carefully with an appropriate heat sealer.

Mason Jars for Preserved Foods: Mason jars are ideal for canning and preserving homegrown or homemade foods. They create a vacuum seal when properly processed, keeping the contents fresh for an extended period. Use various sizes to accommodate different quantities of preserved foods.

Vacuum-Sealed Bags for Perishables: For items like freeze-dried foods, meats, and cheese, vacuum-sealed bags are an excellent choice. These bags remove excess air, preventing oxidation and prolonging the shelf life of the contents. Invest in a vacuum sealer to ensure a secure seal.

Plastic Bins with Lids for Non-Perishables: Large, sturdy plastic bins with tightly fitting lids are perfect for organizing and storing non-perishable items. These bins protect against dust, pests, and light exposure. Label them with the contents and purchase dates for easy identification.

Heavy-Duty Plastic Buckets for Bulk Goods: For storing bulk items like rice, wheat, or sugar, heavy-duty plastic buckets with gamma-seal lids are a solid choice. These buckets provide a durable and pest-resistant storage solution. The gamma-seal lids are easy to open and reseal, ensuring your bulk goods stay fresh.

Freezer Bags for Short-Term Storage: Freezer bags are handy for storing smaller portions of perishable items, like meats and vegetables, in the freezer. They are designed to protect against freezer burn and are resealable, making them a versatile choice for short-term storage needs.

MANAGING SPOILED OR EXPIRED ITEMS

To maintain your food stockpile's quality, it's crucial to understand the factors that can reduce shelf life. The HALT acronym is a useful tool for identifying these enemies of your long-term food storage pantry: Humidity, Air, Light, and Temperature. Additionally, I'll address a fourth risk to your stockpile that you must be on the lookout for as well.

Identifying Spoilage and Safety Disposal

Humidity: Moisture can lead to spoilage and the growth of harmful microorganisms. Use desiccant packs in your storage containers, and store food in a cool, dry place to combat humidity. Consider a dehumidifier for your pantry area.

Air: Oxygen can cause food to deteriorate and become rancid. Vacuum-sealing or using oxygen absorbers can help mitigate this issue. Invest in a quality vacuum sealer to preserve your foods longer.

Light: Exposure to light can degrade the quality of food, leading to nutrient loss and off-flavors. Store your stockpile in a dark area or use opaque containers. Consider using pantry shelves with doors to block out light.

Temperature: Extremes of temperature, both hot and cold, can affect food quality. Maintain a consistent, cool storage temperature to prolong shelf life. Use a thermometer in your storage area to monitor temperature fluctuations.

Pests: Certainly not to be forgotten are insects and rodents! They can infiltrate your food stockpile and really mess things up, or cost you serious time and money. Regularly inspect your storage area for any signs of pests, such as droppings or chewed packaging. Use pest-proof containers and consider placing traps or deterrents in your storage area. Another tip from my experience is if you can keep containers off the ground, such as on a pallet or on a shelf, this is a great first line of defense against many rodents. (although it is not your only line of defense)

To ensure the safety of your family, it's crucial to recognize signs of spoilage such as unusual odors, off-colors, and mold. The CDC reports that foodborne illnesses increase during disasters due to poor sanitation and limited access to fresh food. When you discover spoiled or expired items, follow these steps to safely dispose of them:

Wear protective gear: Use disposable gloves and a mask when handling potentially contaminated items to prevent contact with harmful substances.

Isolate the affected items: Keep them separate from the rest of your stockpile to prevent any potential cross-contamination.

Dispose of them properly: Depending on local regulations, you can compost or bury spoiled items as eco-friendly disposal methods. Ensure they are securely sealed in a container to avoid attracting pests.

Document the loss: Note the items, quantity, and date of disposal for record-keeping purposes. This helps you track inventory changes and financial costs associated with restocking.

REPLENISHING EXPIRED ITEMS

In keeping a well-prepared prepper pantry, renewing expired items is crucial. To maintain the best food stockpile, it's essential to regularly check and replace expired goods. This isn't just a routine; it's about staying ready and ensuring your pantry is reliable. Restocking expired items isn't just swapping things out; it's about keeping your prepper pantry strong and ready for anything that comes your way. Replenishing your stockpile can be cost-effective with the right strategies, let's investigate a few:

Sales and Discounts: Keep an eye out for sales, promotions, and discounts on non-perishable items. Subscribe to store newsletters to stay informed about upcoming deals.

Coupons and Loyalty Programs: Utilize coupons and store loyalty programs to save on prepper pantry essentials. Collect coupons from newspapers, online sources, and store mailers.

Preserve Garden Surplus: If you have a garden, preserve surplus produce through canning or dehydrating to add to your stockpile. Invest in canning equipment and dehydrators for long-term preservation.

Bulk Purchases: Consider bulk purchases for items that have a long shelf life, such as rice, pasta, and canned goods. Buy in larger quantities when prices are favorable and storage space allows.

Trade or Barter: In prepper communities, consider trading or bartering with others for variety and cost savings. Building a network of like-minded individuals can help you access a wider range of products.

Proper storage maintenance and rotation of your food stockpile are essential to ensuring the long-term effectiveness of your prepper pantry. Implementing an inventory system, understanding the enemies of shelf life, recognizing spoilage signs, and replenishing expired items with cost-effective strategies will help you maintain a reliable and well-prepared stockpile.

6

GARDEN CULTIVATION FOR LONG-TERM SUSTAINABILITY: HARVESTING ABUNDANCE, NURTURING SEEDS, AND PRESERVING NATURE'S BOUNTY

"The wise man does at once what the fool does finally."

— BALTASAR GRACIAN

DISCOVER RENEWABLE FOOD SOURCES

In the face of disaster, there are those who panic, and there are those who thrive. Allow me to share an inspiring story of the Anderson family, who faced a catastrophic event with resilience and foresight. While their neighbors struggled, the Anderson's thrived, thanks to their well-prepared approach to survival. Central to their success was the bountiful garden they had cultivated over the years, which complemented their stockpile of essentials. In this chapter, we will explore the vital concept of cultivating long-term sustainability, where we nurture the seeds of self-reliance, harvest abundance, and preserve nature's bounty.

NURTURING YOUR PREPPER PANTRY GARDEN FOR YEARS OF BOUNTY

For a successful food stockpile reserve, integrating a garden is a game-changer. Not only does it supplement your survival strategy, but it also provides fresh, nutrient-rich food. To cultivate a sustainable prepper garden that thrives for years, a strong start is crucial. Begin by evaluating your space—select a well-drained area with access to sunlight, essential for most plants. Test the soil to understand its composition and pH levels, amending it as needed with organic matter or fertilizers to optimize growing conditions. Plan the garden layout efficiently, considering crop rotations, companion planting, and grouping plants with similar water and sunlight needs for effective space utilization.

Invest in quality seeds or starter plants suited for your climate and soil. Start small, gradually expanding as you gain experience. Maintain a diverse crop selection—mix vegetables, herbs, fruits, and perhaps even edible flowers—to maximize yields and foster a self-sustaining ecosystem within your garden.

Regular care to your garden is key to longevity. Implement a consistent watering schedule, ensuring plants receive adequate hydration without waterlogging. Mulch the soil to retain moisture, suppress weeds, and regulate temperature. Inspect plants regularly for pests or diseases, addressing issues promptly to prevent spreading. Consider natural pest control methods and organic fertilizers to maintain a healthy garden ecosystem. You may consider fencing to repel larger animals such as rabbits and deer.

Practice mindful harvesting by picking fruits and vegetables at peak ripeness to encourage continued growth. Save seeds from non-hybrid plants for future planting seasons, creating a sustainable cycle within your garden. Rotate crops annually to prevent soil depletion and pest build-up, supporting long-term garden health.

Lastly, document your garden's progress—keep a journal noting successes, failures, and lessons learned. This information will guide future decisions and improve gardening practices, ensuring a thriving prepper garden for years to come. Now with the basics to your prepper pantry garden captured here are some ideal fruits, vegetables, and herbs that work best for your stockpile garden:

Fruits

Apples: These resilient trees are known for their hardiness. Varieties like Granny Smith and Fuji are excellent choices, offering a balance of sweetness and tartness. With proper storage, apples can last for months, making them a reliable source of vitamin C and dietary fiber. We are blessed to have several apple and pear trees lined outside of our main garden.

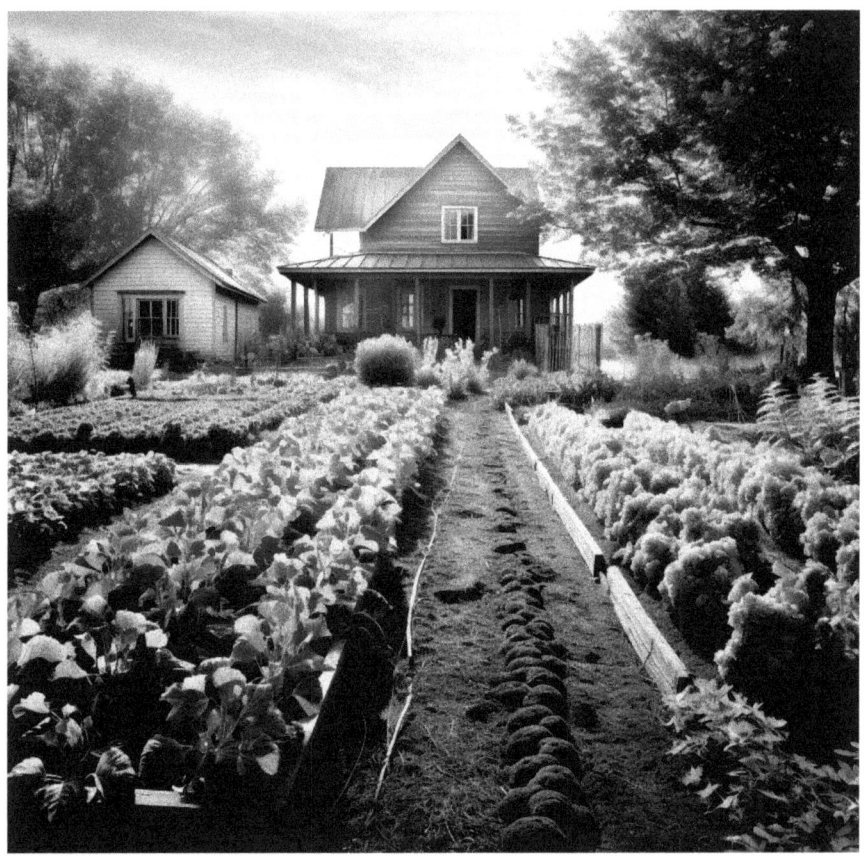

Blueberries: Packed with antioxidants, blueberry bushes are a valuable addition to your garden. Varieties like Blue crop and Chandler yield bountiful harvests. Blueberries can be dehydrated or preserved in jams and jellies for long-term enjoyment.

Strawberries: These versatile plants thrive in various climates and are known for their high yield. Whether you choose June-bearing or Everbearing varieties, strawberries can be frozen, canned, or made into preserves, ensuring a delicious and nutritious treat.

Raspberries: Rich in vitamins and fiber, raspberries are a valuable addition to your garden. Varieties like Heritage and Boyne are known for their resilience. These berries can be frozen, canned, or turned into fruit leather for extended storage.

Vegetables

Tomatoes: One of the most versatile garden staples, tomatoes are essential for your stockpile. Varieties like Roma and San Marzano are ideal for sauces and canning. Tomatoes can be preserved as canned whole, crushed, or diced tomatoes, ensuring you have a base for various dishes.

Carrots: High in vitamins and nutrients, carrots are well-suited for long-term storage. Varieties like Scarlet Nantes and Danvers are reliable choices. Properly stored in a cool, dark place, carrots can last for several months.

Potatoes: Starchy and filling, potatoes are a valuable addition to your stockpile. Varieties like Yukon Gold and Russet Burbank store well in a cool, dark, and dry environment. Properly stored, potatoes can last several months and provide an excellent source of carbohydrates.

Spinach: Rich in vitamins and nutrients, spinach is perfect for fresh consumption and canning. Varieties like Bloomsdale and Space are known for their resilience and adaptability.

Herbs

Basil: Not only a culinary delight but also useful for medicinal purposes. Basil can be harvested, dried, and stored for use in various dishes or herbal remedies.

Oregano: A versatile herb that enhances flavors and has healing properties. Oregano can be dried or used fresh, making it a valuable addition to your garden and kitchen.

Thyme: Adds flavor to dishes and is known for its health benefits. Thyme can be dried or used fresh, infusing your meals with its aromatic essence.

The fruits, vegetables, and herbs listed are by no means an exhaustive selection; they merely serve as a starting point for enhancing a prepper pantry with home-grown produce. The specific crops you choose to cultivate should ideally align with your geographic location. For instance, if you reside in a state like Michigan, growing bananas outdoors might not be a feasible option due to climate constraints. Therefore, it's essential to consider your local climate and soil conditions when tailoring your gardening choices. While this book highlights several common and resilient choices, feel free to diversify your garden with crops that thrive best in your particular area.

Gardening is a rewarding endeavor, but it's not without its challenges, and avoiding common mistakes can make all the difference. Let's look at a few common gardening "rookie mistakes" to avoid for beginners:

ROOKIE MISTAKES GARDENING

Neglecting Soil Quality: Your garden's success hinges on the quality of your soil. Neglecting soil testing and enrichment is a common mistake for beginners. It's essential to invest in good soil preparation by incorporating compost and other organic matter to ensure optimal plant growth.

Overcrowding Plants: New gardeners often underestimate the space plants need to grow. Overcrowding can lead to competition for resources like sunlight, water, and nutrients, stunting growth and reducing overall yield.

Ignoring Pest Management: Pests can quickly decimate your crops. New gardeners often overlook the importance of pest management techniques. Learn to identify and protect your crops from common garden invaders. Employ strategies such as companion planting, which pairs crops that naturally deter pests, and consider using natural pesticides to minimize damage.

Inconsistent Watering: New gardeners may struggle with watering schedules, leading to over or under-watering. Inconsistent watering can stress plants, causing issues like blossom end rot or wilting.

Planting at the Wrong Time: Not understanding plant timelines or disregarding local growing seasons can lead to planting too early or too late. This mistake affects plant development and overall harvest.

For experienced gardeners, here are some "best practices" to enhance your garden's sustainability:

BEST PRACTICES GARDENING

Crop Rotation: Regularly changing the location of crops helps maintain soil fertility and minimizes the risk of disease. Crop rotation is an effective strategy for ensuring long-term soil health. Regularly changing the location of crops is a fundamental practice for maintaining soil fertility and minimizing the risk of disease. Different plants have varying nutrient needs and interactions with the soil. Crop rotation helps balance these factors, preserving your soil's vitality.

Companion Planting: Pairing compatible plant species in close proximity is a strategy employed by experienced gardeners to improve growth and protect against pests. For example, planting tomatoes alongside basil can deter tomato hornworms. Learning which plants work well together and which ones should be kept apart is a valuable skill to maximize the productivity and health of your garden.

Mulching Techniques: Implement effective mulching strategies to conserve moisture, suppress weeds, and regulate soil temperature. Organic mulches like straw or compost provide additional nutrients as they break down.

Integrated Organic Practices: Embrace organic gardening methods by avoiding synthetic chemicals and prioritizing natural fertilizers, composting, and biological pest controls to foster a sustainable garden ecosystem.

Efficient Watering: Water is a precious resource, particularly in a survival scenario. Implement efficient watering methods, such as drip irrigation, sprinklers on a timer, or soaker hoses, to conserve water and ensure your garden's hydration needs are met. Installing a rain barrel system for use in gardening would be a great idea for emergency planning. Gather the rain and use it when needed in your garden.

Seed Vault

Seed saving is a crucial skill for long-term sustainability. Not only does it save you money, but it also ensures a continuous source of crops. Heirloom varieties are particularly valuable since you can replant their seeds. To save seeds effectively, follow these steps:

Harvesting Seeds: When it comes to seed saving, the first step is knowing when and how to harvest seeds from your garden. Seeds should be collected when they are fully mature, which is usually when the plant has reached the end of its growing season. For many vegetables, this means allowing them to ripen on the plant until they are slightly overripe. Fruits like tomatoes should be left on the vine until they're soft and almost ready to eat. When harvesting, use clean and dry hands or tools to avoid introducing moisture that could lead to mold.

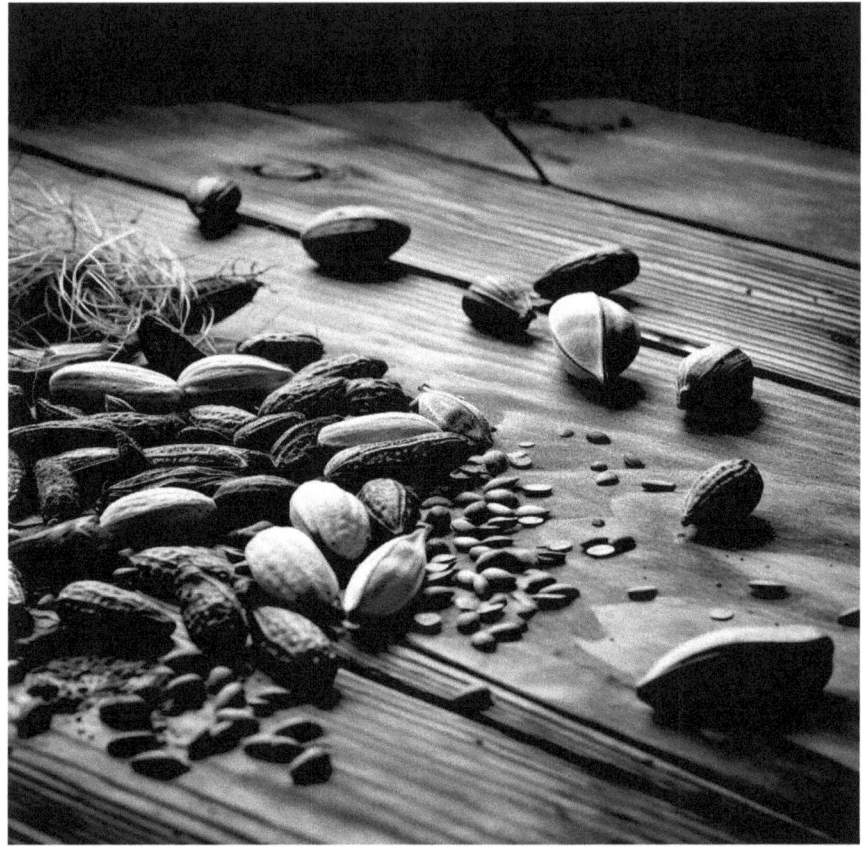

Drying Seeds: Properly drying seeds is essential to prevent mold and ensure their longevity. After harvesting, place the seeds on a clean, dry surface in a well-ventilated area. It's best to use screens or paper towels to avoid seeds sticking together. The goal is to remove as much moisture as possible, which can take anywhere from a few days to a few weeks, depending on the seeds and your local humidity. Ensure that the seeds are completely dry before moving on to the storage phase. You can perform the "snap test" by trying to break a seed with your fingernail; if it snaps cleanly, it's dry enough.

Storage of Seeds: Storing seeds properly is the key to long-term viability. Once your seeds are thoroughly dried, place them in airtight containers, such as glass jars or resealable bags, and label them with the plant type and date of collection. Adding a desiccant, like silica gel, can help absorb any remaining moisture. Store your seeds in a cool, dark, and dry location, such as a refrigerator or a freezer. The goal is to keep the seeds in a state of suspended animation, slowing down their natural aging process. When stored correctly, many seeds can remain viable for several years, allowing you to replant and maintain your garden's self-sufficiency.

Mastering the art of seed saving is a valuable skill that not only ensures the sustainability of your garden, but also empowers you to share seeds with others in your community, fostering a sense of self-reliance and cooperation. By following these steps, you can secure a diverse, long-term food source that is not only cost-effective but also deeply rewarding.

Sustainable protein sources, such as aquaponics and small livestock, complement your garden as well as this amazing prepper pantry you are constructing for your family.

Although these two practices are not for everyone, let's take a closer look at both options.

RAISING SMALL LIVESTOCK

In the context of a 90-day food stockpile, the inclusion of small livestock, such as chickens, rabbits, and quail, offers a valuable source of fresh protein, as well as other essential resources. Integrating these animals into your preparedness plan brings a range of benefits that enhance the quality and sustainability of your stockpile. Here's how raising small livestock can play a crucial role in your 90-day food stockpile strategy:

Protein Source: Small livestock provide a consistent supply of protein-rich food. Chickens offer eggs and meat, while rabbits and quail are excellent sources of lean meat. This variety ensures that you have a renewable protein source, complementing the non-perishable items in your stockpile.

Fresh Food: Small livestock contribute to a steady source of fresh food. Eggs can be collected daily, and rabbits or quail can be harvested as needed, providing a welcome contrast to the preserved and non-perishable items in your stockpile. This fresh food not only improves your diet but also boosts morale during challenging times.

Sound the Alarm: Animals like chickens, ducks, or geese possess acute senses and can react to potential threats, alerting homeowners to unusual activities or disturbances.

Their natural instincts to become agitated or vocalize in response to changes in their environment can serve as an early warning system, providing an extra layer of security against potential dangers.

Resource Recycling: These animals are resourceful recyclers. Chickens, for instance, convert kitchen scraps and garden waste into eggs and manure, which can be used to enrich your garden's soil. This resource utilization promotes a circular economy within your prepper ecosystem, reducing waste and maximizing sustainability.

Self-Sufficiency: By raising small livestock, you become less reliant on external food sources. This self-sufficiency is especially valuable in situations where supply chains may be disrupted or limited. Your ability to breed and raise your animals ensures a consistent protein supply and reinforces your resilience.

Education and Skill Development: Raising small livestock equips you with knowledge and skills in animal care and management, which can be invaluable not only for your immediate needs, but also as a barterable skill in a community of preppers. Sharing this expertise fosters a sense of cooperation and mutual support among neighbors.

Manure for Gardening: The manure produced by chickens, rabbits, and quail is a rich source of fertilizer for your garden. Utilizing this natural resource enhances your gardening efforts, contributing to higher yields and healthier crops. In a 90-day stockpile scenario, this gardening support can be essential for supplementing your food supplies.

Compact Space Usage: Small livestock can be raised in relatively small spaces, making them suitable for urban and suburban preppers. Chicken coops, rabbit hutches, and quail enclosures can be designed to fit various settings, ensuring that you can raise animals even with limited land.

To incorporate small livestock into your 90-day food stockpile strategy, you'll need to set up appropriate housing, provide proper nutrition, and understand the specific needs of each type of animal. These crucial components are not covered in this book, feel free to explore this on your own if you decide that raising livestock is a fit for your family. It's an investment in time and resources, but the rewards are substantial, ensuring a well-rounded, resilient, and sustainable approach to food security.

Aquaponics

While not for everyone, aquaponics systems combine fish farming with plant cultivation, creating a closed-loop system that produces both protein and vegetables. The fish waste provides valuable nutrients for the plants, which in turn filter the water for the fish. To incorporate aquaponics into your 90-day food stockpile strategy, you'll need to acquire the necessary equipment and understand the basics of system setup, fish care, and plant cultivation. It's an investment in both time and resources, but the rewards are significant, ensuring a more comprehensive, resilient, and nutritious stockpile. This efficient system offers a sustainable source of both protein and fresh produce for your family.

Continuous Food Production: One of the primary benefits of aquaponics is its ability to provide a consistent source of food year-round. In a 90-day food stockpile scenario, this means a continuous supply of fresh vegetables and fish, significantly extending the variety of nutrients available to you and your family.

Efficient Resource Utilization: Aquaponics maximizes resource efficiency. The waste produced by fish becomes a nutrient-rich fertilizer for plants, creating a closed-loop system. It reduces water usage compared to traditional gardening, making it a sustainable option even in times of limited water availability.

Versatile Crop Choices: With aquaponics, you can grow a wide range of vegetables and herbs, allowing you to diversify your diet. Leafy greens like lettuce and kale, as well as herbs such as basil and cilantro, flourish in aquaponic systems. This variety enhances your nutritional options during an emergency.

Protein Source: The fish component of aquaponics provides a consistent protein source. Tilapia, catfish, and trout are commonly used in these systems. With proper care, these fish can thrive and reproduce, ensuring a sustainable protein source for your 90-day food stockpile.

Space Efficiency: Aquaponic systems can be adapted to fit various spaces, including small backyards, patios, or even indoor settings. This versatility makes them accessible to urban and suburban preppers, enabling them to cultivate food in limited areas.

Resilience in Uncertain Times: In a crisis, traditional food supplies may be disrupted. Aquaponics offers a level of self-sufficiency that can be crucial during emergencies. The reliability of this system ensures that, even when other food sources are scarce, you can continue to harvest fresh produce and fish.

Learning and Adaptation: Building and maintaining an aquaponic system also equips you with valuable knowledge and skills in sustainable food production. This knowledge can be shared with your community, strengthening bonds and promoting self-reliance among neighbors.

While aquaponics can't replace all the components of a well-rounded food stockpile, it serves as a vital supplement. By combining aquaponics and gardening with traditional prepper pantry items you create a robust and diversified approach to food security that significantly enhances your preparedness for any situation.

Hunting, Fishing, Foraging

In the quest for long-term sustainability, integrating hunting, fishing, and foraging into your self-sufficient lifestyle offers an array of benefits beyond mere survival. These skills provide a deeper connection to nature, foster a sense of self-reliance, and broaden your food sources. Depending on your region, various wild game, fish, and edible plants are available. Equip yourself with the right tools for each, let's explore:

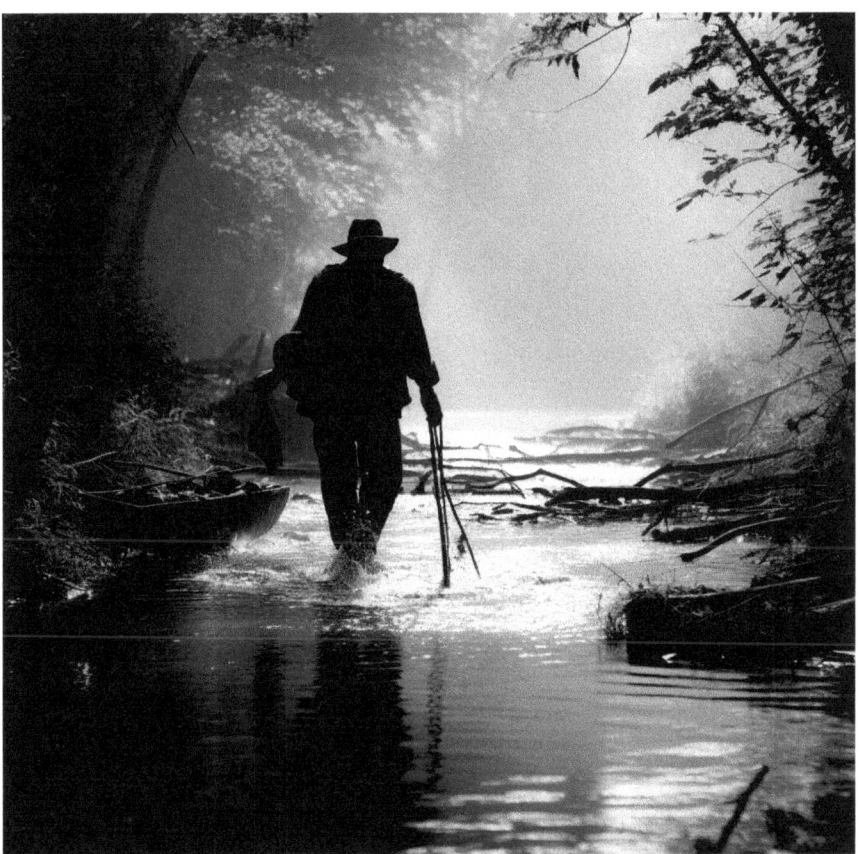

Hunting: Hunting is not merely a means of acquiring meat; it's a profound connection to the primal instinct of self-sufficiency. Whether you're pursuing game such as deer, turkey, or small game like squirrels and rabbits, hunting instills patience, discipline, and a profound appreciation for the circle of life. The rewards are plentiful, with a varied source of protein that can supplement your diet for months. Understanding your local hunting regulations, the best hunting seasons, and the behavior of your prey is essential for success.

Hunting weapons: Rifles, shotguns, and bows are essential tools for hunting game. Ensure you have a thorough understanding of local hunting regulations and practices.

Fishing: Fishing extends your self-sufficiency to the waters, providing a rich source of protein and a calming, meditative experience. Learning the art of angling is not limited to catching fish; it includes understanding the ecosystems of local water bodies, knowing the types of fish available, and mastering various fishing techniques. From freshwater species like bass, trout, and catfish to saltwater catches such as salmon and flounder, fishing offers both a recreational and survival advantage. Moreover, fish can be smoked, dried, or canned, allowing for long-term storage.

Fishing equipment: Fishing rods, reels, and bait are essential for different fishing environments. Learn the best fishing techniques for your location and target species.

Foraging: Foraging brings you closer to the land, immersing you in the rich tapestry of wild edibles. Whether you're picking dandelions, cattails, chickweed, or violets, foraging is a lesson in resourcefulness and adaptability. It offers a diverse palette of flavors and nutrients, enhancing your diet while reducing your reliance on cultivated crops. Additionally, foraging helps you connect with the natural world, teaching you to recognize seasonal changes, identify edible plants, and learn from the wisdom of nature. The berries and herbs you gather depend on your region, but they include a wide array of species such as blackberries, raspberries, and wild strawberries.

The top 10 wild edibles include dandelion, cattail, chickweed, violets, wild garlic, lambs quarters, plantain, wood sorrel, purslane, and nettles. These wild edibles offer variety and essential nutrients, complementing your diet.

Foraging requires some specialized equipment to gather and process wild edibles. Basic equipment includes:

Wildcrafting bags or baskets: Used for collecting wild edibles without damaging them.

Plant identification guides: Essential for recognizing edible species and avoiding harmful plants.

Pocket knife: Useful for harvesting plants and processing edibles.

Drying and storage equipment: Suitable for preserving collected edibles.

Understanding the specific tools, equipment, and techniques for each type of game or plant ensures that you can take full advantage of the resources around you. As you become proficient in hunting, fishing, and foraging, you're not only securing sustenance for your family, but also forging a profound connection to the natural world. These skills embody the essence of self-reliance, ensuring that you're prepared not only for short-term survival but for the flourishing of your self-sustaining lifestyle.

Remember that as you embrace these methods of sourcing food, always respect local regulations, ethical hunting and fishing practices, and sustainable foraging guidelines to preserve the balance of nature and ensure a lasting source of nourishment for yourself and your community.

Permaculture

Permaculture is an ecological design system that emphasizes sustainable living, ethical resource management, and harmonious coexistence with nature. It aligns perfectly with the principles of a 90-day prepper pantry survival stockpile, as it offers a holistic approach to long-term sustainability and self-reliance. In the spirit of permaculture, we embrace principles like "people care," "earth care," and "fair share." During a crisis, your food and gear stockpile can positively impact your local community. Sharing surplus food or essential items can foster cooperation, ensuring a safer, more resilient environment for all. By adopting these principles, we prepare not just for ourselves but for the well-being of our neighbors as well.

Here's how you can connect permaculture principles to your survival stockpile guide:

People Care: In the context of a prepper pantry, "people care" involves prioritizing the well-being and preparedness of your family and community. It encourages self-reliance, holistic well-being, and supportive relationships within communities. Permaculture promotes education, access to resources, and creating systems that meet human needs while respecting environmental limits. By prioritizing the welfare of individuals and communities, this principle ensures sustainable living practices that support long-term resilience.

Earth Care: This principle emphasizes responsible stewardship of the Earth. It involves nurturing and regenerating natural systems, fostering biodiversity, and minimizing environmental impact. Practices include conservation, organic gardening, water harvesting, and regenerative agriculture. By understanding and respecting natural patterns, permaculture promotes harmony with the land, aiming to leave it healthier and more productive than before.

Fair Share: Fair Share involves equitable distribution and sharing of resources. It emphasizes the idea of using only what is needed, conserving surpluses, and reinvesting them back into the system. This principle encourages responsible consumption, ethical business practices, and fair distribution of resources among individuals and communities. Fair Share also advocates for giving back to the Earth, acknowledging our interconnectedness with the planet and other living beings.

Connecting permaculture to a book on a 90-day prepper pantry survival stockpile involves implementing its core principles in food production, resource management, and community support. By integrating permaculture into the survival plan, you not only ensure the availability of food and resources in times of crisis but also create a resilient, self-sustaining environment for the long haul.

In the journey of crafting a 90-day prepper pantry survival stockpile, this chapter has been a vital stepping stone, guiding you through the intricacies of cultivating long-term sustainability. As we conclude, it's clear that self-reliance goes far beyond mere survival – it's about creating a thriving, resilient future for yourself and your community. By exploring renewable food sources, you've learned to harness the potential of a well-planned garden, yielding a diverse range of fruits, vegetables, and herbs that not only nourish but also provide a profound connection to the land. The art of seed saving and heirloom varieties empowers you to maintain the cycle of life in your garden, ensuring the legacy of bountiful harvests. This knowledge is your insurance for long-term sustainability, safeguarding your ability to put food in the ground to complement your stockpile inside your home. Hunting, fishing, and foraging, while critical for sourcing protein and wild edibles, offer more than sustenance. They instill a deep connection to nature, cultivating patience, resilience, and an appreciation for the cycle of life. The benefits extend beyond your pantry; they extend to your spirit and your place in the natural world. Permaculture principles—people care, earth care, and fair share—encourage you to think beyond your immediate needs. They beckon you to foster a sense of community, ensuring that your knowledge and resources benefit not just your family but also your neighbors. The stockpile you've built is not just a personal safety net; it's a potential lifeline for those around you. By sharing knowledge, supporting one another, and tending to the earth, you're not only safeguarding your future, but also nurturing a community of strength and resilience.

7

GUARDING YOUR GOODS: STRATEGIES FOR SECURING AND CONCEALING YOUR 90-DAY STOCKPILE

"In every adversity, there lies the seed of an equivalent advantage."

— NAPOLEON HILL

MAINTAINING OPERATIONAL SECURITY OF YOUR STOCKPILE

I n the midst of chaos and crisis, the prepared thrive, and their success hinges on more than just having a well-stocked pantry. A key element of survival is guarding your goods against potential threats. Picture this: a family well-versed in the art of prepping and fully stocked with essential supplies. When disaster strikes, they not only weather the storm but protect their home and the precious contents within. In this chapter, we will delve into the strategies and practices that ensure the protection of your 90-day stockpile, securing your family's survival in the face of adversity.

Concealment and Camouflage Techniques for Your Stockpile

Concealment is an art every prepper should master. We will explore the secrets of hiding your supplies in plain sight. You will discover various methods to keep your stockpile safe and hidden from prying eyes. Proper concealment can mean the difference between abundance and deprivation during a crisis.

The Low Profile Advantage

Maintaining a low profile is the first rule of prepping. To protect your stockpile, you must minimize your exposure to potential threats. Learn to blend seamlessly into your community, and avoid drawing attention to your preparations. Bragging about your stockpile or displaying conspicuous prepper gear should be avoided at all costs. Personally, I take the time inside my garage to break down any boxes of prepping equipment or weapons purchased. The boxes get cut up, or folded, and placed directly into the recycle dumpster. I try at all costs to not let manufacturer labeled boxes (outside of generic Amazon boxes) sit exposed at the street corner on trash day advertising to everyone my fancy new purchases. Another real-life concealment situation is I have 2 very large shrubs planted around each of my 2 rainwater collection drums so as to not show them off to the world. Yes, people can see them if they look hard enough and snoop around, just don't broadcast things that are unnecessary is my point here. The foundation of operational security begins with discretion.

STRATEGIC PLACEMENT AND CAMOUFLAGE

Concealing your stockpile within your home is a skill every prepper should master. Learn the art of spreading your supplies throughout your living space, avoiding the risk of losing everything in one fell swoop. Whether it's blending storage containers with common household items, hiding supplies behind seemingly mundane structures, or utilizing color and pattern strategies for effective concealment, camouflage adds an extra layer of security to your prepper toolkit. This section explores options for dividing your goods into multiple caches, ensuring that you'll always have access to vital resources, even if one area is compromised.

Hidden Compartments: Install hidden compartments within existing furniture or fixtures in your home, such as false bottoms in cabinets or hidden drawers in closets. Utilize these concealed spaces to store smaller, valuable items or emergency supplies discreetly. Your home can be like Hogwarts! Sorry if you've never read the Harry Potter series, but what rock are you living under if you've never heard of the magical Hogwarts Castle from this epic tale?

Clever Shelving: Create shelving units with adjustable panels or secret compartments. These can be disguised as regular shelves but can hide items behind or within them, providing both storage and camouflage. There are many useful benefits here when it comes to quick access to firearms, hidden in plain sight!

Underfloor Storage: If feasible, consider creating under-floor storage spaces. Lift up a section of flooring to reveal a hidden storage area where you can stash larger supplies or emergency kits. Ensure the access point is well-concealed with a rug or furniture.

Camouflaged Furniture: Invest in furniture designed with built-in storage that doesn't look like traditional storage. For instance, a coffee table with a hidden compartment or an ottoman that doubles as a storage chest can blend seamlessly into your living space.

False Walls or Panels: Construct false walls or panels that blend into the existing structure of your home. These can hide storage spaces behind them, making it challenging for anyone to detect the presence of your stockpile.

Customized Closets: Optimize your closet space by customizing it to include hidden shelves or compartments. Install false backs in closets or create additional shelving systems that can be easily concealed by clothing or other items.

Repurposed Furniture: Use repurposed furniture with built-in storage. Old wardrobes, armoires, or even vintage cabinets can be adapted to conceal your prepping supplies while maintaining a functional and aesthetically pleasing appearance.

Decoy Items: Integrate decoy items or containers that mimic everyday household objects. For instance, use false book spines to create a concealed storage area on a bookshelf or hide supplies within containers that resemble cleaning products. I know a person who stocks canned food under their kitchen sink.

Wall Art Concealment: Transform wall art into functional concealment. Install artwork that opens to reveal hidden storage spaces behind, providing both a decorative element and a practical means of hiding your prepping supplies.

Ceiling Concealment: Explore the possibility of ceiling storage. Suspended storage compartments or racks can be hidden above eye level and accessed through retractable ladders or pulley systems, offering an unconventional yet effective concealment solution.

Mastering the art of concealing your prepping stockpile within your home involves a thoughtful combination of strategic placement and creative camouflage. By implementing these ingenious ideas, preppers can not only safeguard their essential supplies effectively but also seamlessly integrate preparedness into their living spaces, ensuring both security and practicality in times of need.

LEGAL CONSIDERATIONS

Prepping exists within the bounds of the law today, but what if those bounds were to change drastically in an apocalyptic scenario? In this section, we discuss the importance of understanding the legal landscape in your region. While we always advocate for compliance with existing laws, we also explore the realities of survival when societal structures break down. Knowing your rights and responsibilities is vital for maintaining security and ensuring your stockpile remains protected.

Local Laws and Regulations: Understand the existing laws and regulations related to prepping, firearms, and self-defense in your local area.

State Laws: Familiarize yourself with state-level legislation that may affect your prepping activities, such as firearm ownership and storage regulations.

Federal Laws: Be aware of federal laws that govern certain aspects of prepping, including firearm purchases and transfer requirements.

Compliance: Always strive to stay in compliance with the law. This includes proper licensing, permits, and adherence to storage regulations.

Zoning Regulations: Check zoning regulations that pertain to your property, especially if you plan on burying caches or setting up structures for prepping purposes.

Potential Changes: Consider the possibility of legal changes during a crisis or disaster scenario. Understand how these changes might impact your prepping activities.

Legal Documentation: Keep important legal documents related to your prepping, such as permits, licenses, and firearm ownership records, in a secure and accessible location.

Consult Legal Experts: When in doubt, seek legal advice from experts who specialize in prepping and self-defense laws.

Remember that legal considerations may vary depending on your location and the evolving nature of the situation, so staying informed and seeking professional guidance is crucial.

FIREARMS FOR SELF-DEFENSE

Firearms are valuable tools for self-defense, but they come with significant responsibilities. I could make this an entire book, however in an ultimate prepper pantry guide I will limit this to a section. You'll learn about some of the most common types of firearms, their respective advantages, and their potential role in protecting your family.

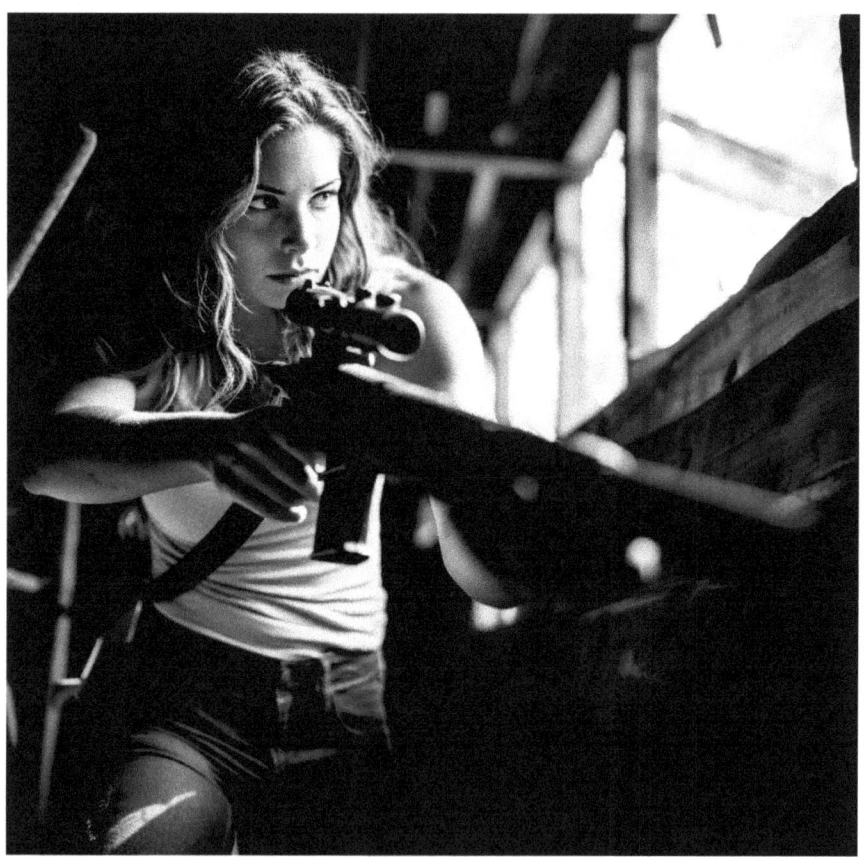

Popular Firearms for Self-Defense:

Handguns: Compact and versatile, handguns like the Glock 19 or Smith & Wesson M&P Shield are popular choices for self-defense due to their ease of use, concealability, and widespread availability.

Shotguns: Shotguns, such as the Remington 870 or Mossberg 500, are valued for their stopping power and versatility in home defense scenarios. Their intimidation factor can act as a deterrent.

Modern Sporting Rifles: AR-15 style rifles, like the Colt AR-15 or Ruger AR-556, are appreciated for their accuracy and customization options, making them effective for both home defense and potential survival situations.

Responsible Firearm Ownership:

Secure Storage: Store firearms securely in a gun safe or lockbox to prevent unauthorized access. Responsible ownership includes ensuring that guns are inaccessible to children, visitors, or individuals without proper training.

Compliance with Laws: Adhere to local, state, and federal firearm laws to maintain responsible ownership. This includes obtaining necessary permits, undergoing background checks, and staying informed about any legal requirements related to firearms.

Regular Maintenance: Regularly maintain and clean firearms to ensure their proper functioning. Responsible owners understand the importance of routine inspections and upkeep to guarantee the reliability of their weapons.

FIREARMS TRAINING AND SAFETY:

Training Programs: Engage in comprehensive firearms training programs to develop proficiency in handling and shooting. Seek courses that cover not only marksmanship but also emphasize situational awareness, decision-making, and safe firearm manipulation.

Regular Practice: Practice regularly at a shooting range to maintain and enhance your shooting skills. Consistent practice fosters muscle memory, improving your ability to handle firearms effectively and safely in high-stress situations.

Safety Protocols: Prioritize safety by following fundamental protocols, including keeping the firearm pointed in a safe direction, treating every gun as if it's loaded, and maintaining proper trigger discipline. A commitment to safety is integral to responsible firearms use in a prepping context.

SELF-DEFENSE STRATEGIES

When all else fails and your family's safety is at stake, self-defense becomes paramount. In this section, the topics covered are the importance of self-defense, responsible firearm ownership, and the knowledge and skills you need to keep your loved ones safe. Understanding self-defense strategies is a fundamental aspect of prepping. Here are a few that can keep your family, and that survival stockpile, protected like Fort Knox.

Personal Security Training: Engage in self-defense and personal security training to build essential skills in protecting yourself and your loved ones. Attend classes or workshops that cover basic techniques, situational awareness, and effective communication to enhance your ability to handle potential threats. Mastering the fundamentals of self-defense provides a strong foundation for prepping by empowering individuals to navigate uncertain situations with confidence.

Home Security Measures: Strengthen your home security with practical measures such as reinforcing doors and windows, installing motion sensor lighting, and utilizing security cameras. Ensure that your residence is well-lit and visible, deterring potential intruders. Additionally, establish a clear communication plan with family members to coordinate responses in case of emergencies, and consider investing in a reliable home security system for added protection.

Self-Defense Tools: Equip yourself with appropriate self-defense tools that align with legal regulations and personal comfort levels. This may include items such as pepper spray, personal alarms, or tactical flashlights. Familiarize yourself with the proper usage of these tools and incorporate them into your everyday carry items. Additionally, consider exploring self-defense tools like non-lethal weapons or, where legally permissible, firearms, ensuring proper training and adherence to local laws to responsibly integrate them into your prepping strategy.

We will also explore the principles of personal safety, situational awareness, and conflict avoidance. You'll learn how to recognize and respond to potential threats, as well as effective ways to de-escalate situations without resorting to violence.

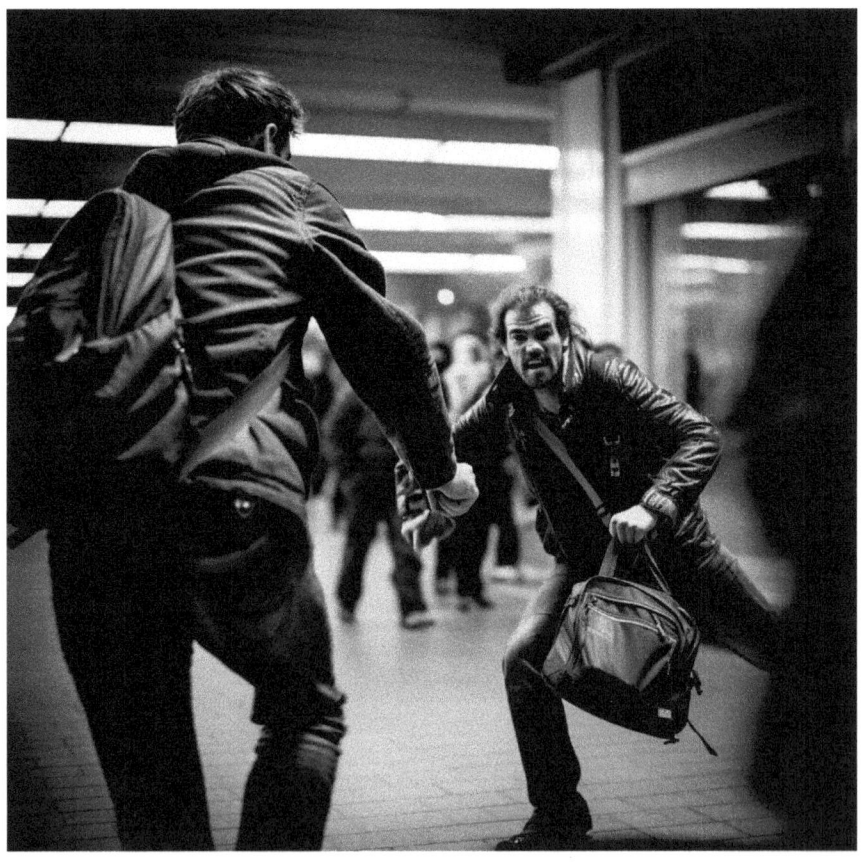

PERSONAL SAFETY

Threat Assessment: Begin with a comprehensive evaluation of potential threats in your environment. This includes identifying high-crime areas in your region, recognizing potential hazards within your home, and understanding the risks associated with daily activities.

Risk Mitigation: Implement measures to reduce risks. This may involve reinforcing your home's security, taking precautions when traveling through risky areas, and securing your stockpile against theft or intrusion with locks or alarms.

Emergency Plans: Develop emergency plans that cater to various scenarios, such as home invasions, natural disasters, or civil unrest. Ensure every family member is familiar with these plans and knows their role in an emergency. Practicing helps ease everyone's mind and it can be a fun family activity. Turn off the TV, go run a simulated fire drill with the kids, and see what happens.

SITUATIONAL AWARENESS

Constant Vigilance: Stay alert and aware of your surroundings at all times. This means avoiding distractions like excessive smartphone use or headphone reliance when in public spaces. If you have one of the larger shelf-stable food stashes around and word gets out, your family could quickly become a target.

Recognizing Anomalies: Train yourself to identify unusual behaviors or situations that might signal a threat. Pay attention to people's body language, sudden crowd movements, or any signs of danger. Loitering vehicles or new people tend to stand out. It's your job to identify this strange activity and at the very least prepare your family.

Risk Assessment: Continuously assess the level of risk in your environment. Is it safe to proceed down a particular street, enter a building, or interact with a stranger? Situational awareness empowers you to make informed decisions based on your surroundings.

CONFLICT AVOIDANCE

De-Escalation: When faced with a potential conflict, the first goal is to de-escalate the situation. Try to defuse tensions through verbal communication, maintaining a calm demeanor, and showing empathy towards others.

Escape Routes: Always be aware of possible escape routes in any location you're in. This proactive approach provides a quick means of removing yourself and your loved ones from danger.

Avoiding Confrontation: Steer clear of situations that may escalate into violence. This includes walking away from arguments, refraining from engaging with aggressive individuals, and prioritizing personal safety over ego. This is important to practice and preach to your children as well.

Conflict Resolution: If conflict becomes inevitable, employ conflict resolution skills that prioritize minimal harm. The objective should be to protect yourself while avoiding harm to others whenever possible.

INTEGRATION INTO YOUR PREPPING STRATEGY

Self-defense and firearm ownership should be integral parts of your overall prepping strategy. Prepping isn't just about survival; it's also about maintaining your moral compass. The ethical considerations of self-defense with a firearm emphasize the importance of preserving life whenever possible and using force only as a last resort. Learning how to seamlessly integrate self-defense measures, firearms, and safety protocols into your preparedness plan to ensure your family's well-being during challenging times will increase your odds in a world when your 90-day food stockpile will be needed. Stay Vigilant my friends!

In the unpredictable world of prepping, guarding your goods isn't just about keeping your pantry safe; it's about ensuring your family's safety. By understanding and implementing these strategies, you're well on your way to thriving in any catastrophe, no matter how dire the circumstances may seem. Your 90-day stockpile will remain protected, providing a lifeline during times of crisis.

8

THE PSYCHOLOGY OF PREPAREDNESS: MANAGING A POSITIVE PREPPER MINDSET IN YOUR PANTRY PLAN

"When the time to perform arrives, the time to prepare has passed."

— HORACE

A BATTLE-TESTED APPROACH TO POSITIVITY

In the hallowed halls of military lore, stories echo of soldiers maintaining a Positive Mental Attitude (PMA) amid the chaos of battle. Consider the tale of Sergeant James Mitchell, a U.S. Marine thrust into the crucible of uncertainty during a mission in WWII. Amid the threat of survival and with limited provisions, Mitchell's unwavering positive mindset not only steered him through adversity, but also uplifted the morale of his unit. In 1944, Mitchell's courageous and selfless actions earned him the prestigious Navy Cross.

What can preppers glean from such tales as we navigate the psychological terrain of preparedness, specifically within the context of our pantry plan? There lies an invaluable lesson in cultivating a resilient positive mental attitude (PMA) amidst the uncertainties, a mindset capable of fortifying us through the psychological terrain of readiness.

UNDERSTANDING THE PSYCHOLOGICAL IMPACT OF A CRISIS

The psychology of preparedness is a critical aspect of survival during catastrophic events. The human response to fear, anxiety, and stress is as integral to survival as the stockpile itself. Recognizing these emotional responses allows preppers to implement proactive coping strategies. Research underscores that individuals armed with a positive mindset in times of crisis are not only more adaptable, but also better equipped to make rational decisions. Yes, even when discussing an Ultimate Survival Pantry we need to mention your mindset. It's not just about having the necessary supplies; it's about cultivating the right attitude to ensure effective decision-making and resilience. I've touched on the topic of positive mental attitude (PMA) in several of my other book's as I feel one's mental makeup is more important than their physical state in a worst-case scenario event. Things will break, things will go wrong, people will let you down, family may get sick or worse. Ok, now what? Your attitude and adaptability are paramount to increasing your family's odds of survival.

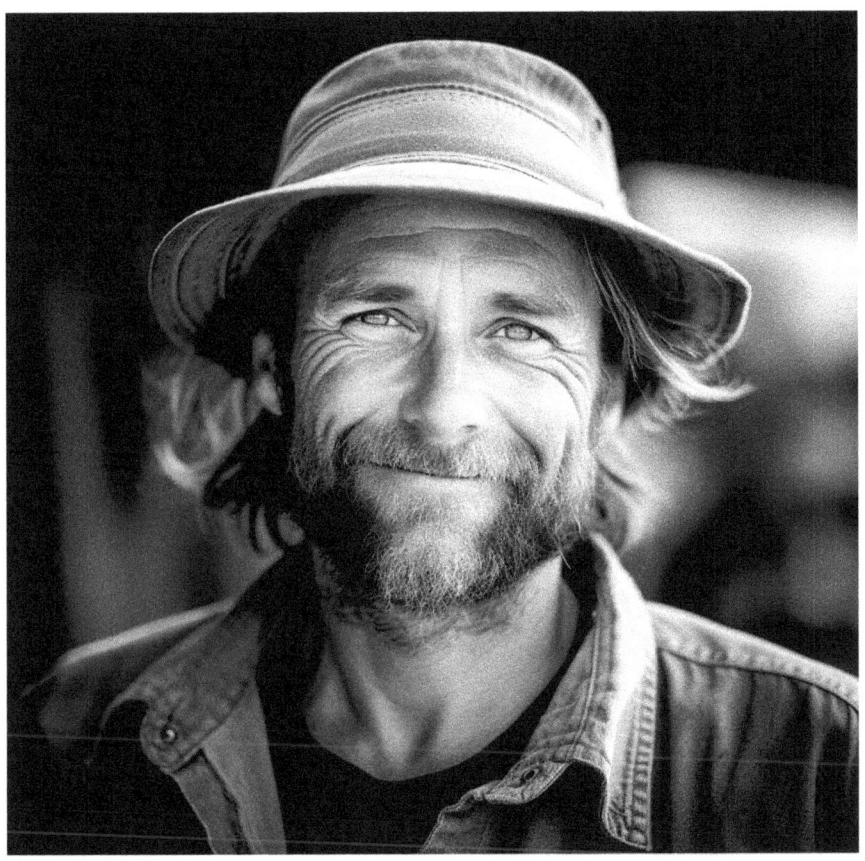

MAINTAIN A POSITIVE MENTAL ATTITUDE (PMA)

Positivity and hope are powerful psychological tools. During a crisis, these tools might as well be under a magnifying glass! Maintaining a positive attitude can help your family cope with the stress and uncertainty of disaster situations. Focusing on what you can control, rather than dwelling on what you can't, will greatly enhance your resilience. This is not a "self-help" book in the Tony Robbins sort of way, but positive self-talk is so very important. Again, if you are relying on your food reserves, something has gone wrong. How that voice in your head communicates with you will impact how you handle the situations that come next.

Positivity also fosters a sense of unity among family members, encouraging mutual support. A positive outlook can inspire creative solutions, such as turning adversity into an opportunity for growth and learning. For those of you with young kids around, they are absorbing everything you do, just like a sponge. I have 4 children at home myself, so this is seen each day by my wife and I. Think more, say less, talk nice to yourself, your actions will have consequences both good and bad.

BUILDING A POSITIVE MINDSET

Encouraging a positive mindset involves more than crisis management—it's about embracing the prepping lifestyle. Celebrate small victories and milestones to maintain enthusiasm. Positivity should permeate the entire prepper journey, turning preparedness into a shared adventure rather than a burdensome duty.

Cultivate a Sense of Accomplishment: Break down your prepping goals into smaller, achievable tasks. Completing these tasks provides a sense of accomplishment and reinforces the idea that you are making progress.

Celebrate Preparedness Milestones: Whether it's reaching a certain quantity of stored food or successfully conducting a family drill, take the time to acknowledge and celebrate these achievements. This fosters a positive atmosphere within your prepper community.

Foster a Learning Environment: Embrace the mindset of continuous improvement. Encourage your family to learn new skills related to prepping, whether it's mastering a new cooking technique or understanding the principles of water purification.

Engage in Group Discussions: Regularly discuss the importance of your prepper pantry and the role it plays in ensuring the family's safety. Open dialogue helps in addressing concerns, fostering understanding, and promoting a shared commitment to the prepping lifestyle.

Optimism Amid Challenges: Approach challenges as opportunities for growth. Whether it's a temporary shortage or a failed gardening experiment, maintain an optimistic perspective and view setbacks as valuable lessons in the journey toward self-sufficiency.

EXAMPLES FROM HISTORY: PSYCHOLOGICAL IMPACT OF CRISIS

The Great Depression: During the Great Depression, families faced economic hardship and scarcity. Those who maintained a positive outlook and adapted their lifestyles were more resilient in the face of adversity. Learning from this era, preppers today can appreciate the value of flexibility and a positive mindset when resources are scarce.

Cuban Missile Crisis: The Cuban Missile Crisis brought the world to the brink of nuclear war. Families and individuals who had prepared emotionally for the possibility of conflict demonstrated remarkable resilience. The crisis highlighted the importance of mental preparedness alongside physical preparations.

Hurricane Katrina: The aftermath of Hurricane Katrina demonstrated the psychological toll of a natural disaster. Individuals and communities that focused on collective strength and mutual support showcased the importance of a positive mindset in navigating the challenging aftermath of a crisis. As Louisianans commenced the process of rebuilding their lives, maintaining a positive mindset became pivotal for their future in the aftermath of the catastrophic event that was Hurricane Katrina.

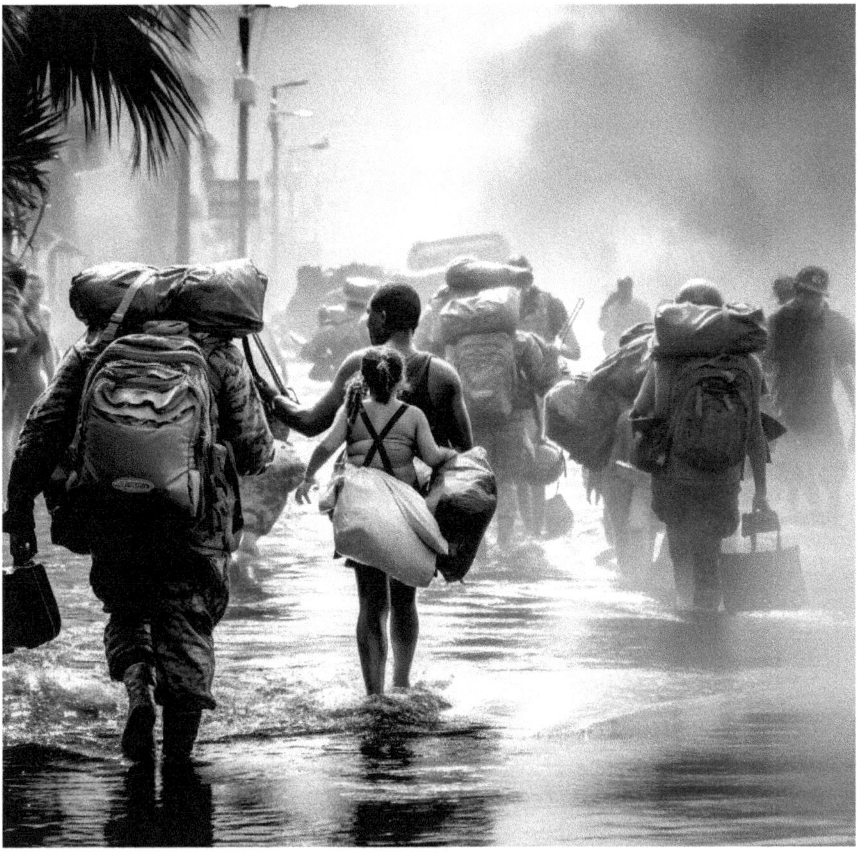

KNOWLEDGE AND TRAINING

Education and training are essential components of the prepper mindset. Knowing how to use your tools, administer first aid, and navigate challenging situations instills confidence. When you and your family understand what to do in an emergency, fear diminishes, and rational problem-solving becomes more accessible. Regularly practice survival skills, conduct fire drills, and stay updated on the latest information related to disaster preparedness in your area. Training sessions can help family members become familiar with various tools, from the proper use of a fire extinguisher to effective communication during a crisis. You likely have in your pantry the components to concoct several helpful, possibly even life-saving, herbal remedies with a clear head on your shoulders.

Flexibility

Preparedness is not about rigid adherence to a single plan; it's about adaptability. Disaster scenarios rarely unfold exactly as expected. Being prepared for change and ready to adjust plans on the fly is a hallmark of a successful prepper mindset. What if pests get into your "sealed" flour when going to make bread? You can stew about it and let it ruin your day, or you can brush it off and move on. Of course I'm suggesting you fix the problem, so as to not let it get out of hand, but repeating to yourself something like "It's not my fault. A situation like this could have happened to anyone. Survivorman himself, Les Stroud could have pests in his food stockpile!" Flexible, positive self-talk will help your perspective and mood here. Do not beat yourself up. Find the pest source, fix the problem, move on to making delicious bread for your family!

In real-life emergencies, circumstances can shift rapidly. The ability to change course when needed and improvise solutions with available resources is invaluable. Embracing flexibility reduces anxiety and empowers you to overcome unexpected challenges.

Stay Informed

Accurate and up-to-date information is a powerful tool during a crisis. Whether you're monitoring weather conditions, keeping an eye on potential threats, or staying informed about local resources and relief efforts, reliable information is essential for making informed decisions. This is as much about keeping your brain sharp, as it is about keeping your communication lines up.

Having access to news sources, emergency alerts, and communication devices is critical. It allows you to track developments and adapt your strategy as the situation unfolds. Preparedness isn't solely about stockpiling; it's about staying informed and making well-informed decisions.

Community Building

In times of crisis, a supportive community of like-minded individuals or families becomes a crucial asset. Just as in business, where the quality of your connections shapes your success, the same principle applies to preparedness. Collaborating with others not only brings diverse perspectives, but also enhances safety measures and resourcefulness, making challenging situations more manageable.

Building a prepper community can involve sharing knowledge, resources, and responsibilities. Neighbors or friends with complementary skills can be invaluable allies during a crisis. Collective efforts can also enhance security by establishing a support system for all members involved.

In each of these situations, having a well-prepared stockpile can provide both physical sustenance and peace of mind. Food stockpiling empowers individuals and families to take control of their well-being during crises, offering a lifeline when traditional support systems break down.

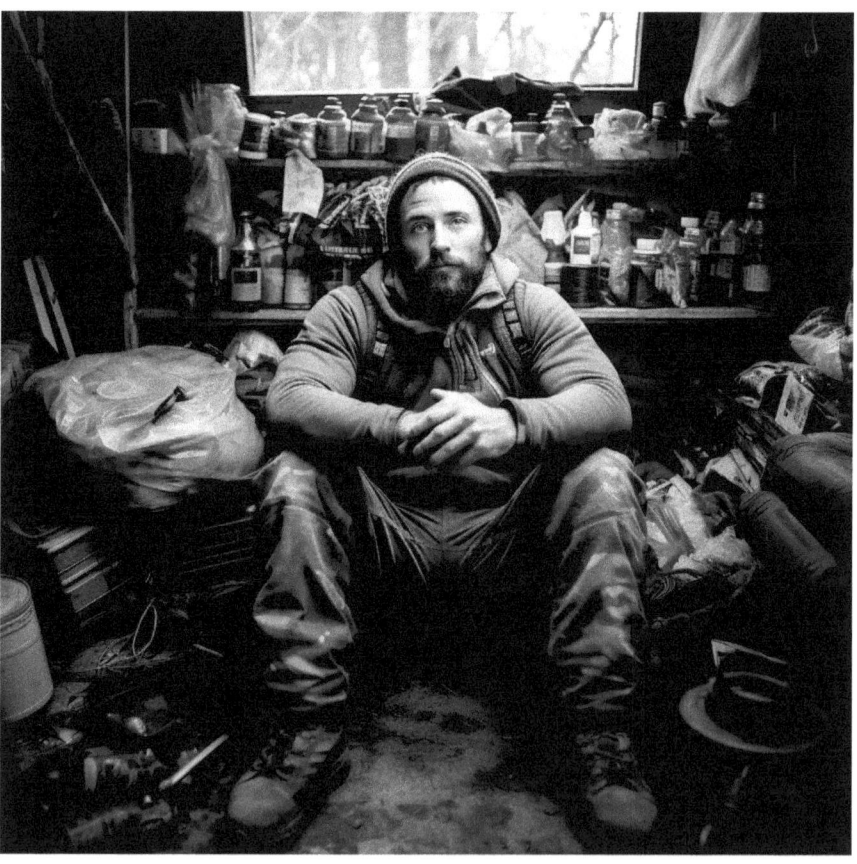

COPING WITH STRESS AND ANXIETY

The ability to manage stress is foundational to maintaining a positive prepper mindset. Techniques such as mindfulness, deep breathing exercises, and adherence to a routine can significantly diminish stress levels. Acknowledging that stress is an inevitable part of the prepping journey lays the groundwork for building resilience over the long term.

Mindfulness Practices: Incorporate mindfulness techniques into your daily routine. Whether it's meditation, deep breathing exercises, or moments of intentional focus, mindfulness can help center your thoughts and alleviate stress.

Establish a Prepping Routine: Structure your prepping activities into a routine. Knowing that you have dedicated time for planning, inventory checks, and drills can reduce the anxiety associated with uncertainty.

Regularly Review and Update the Plans: Feeling in control is crucial for preppers. Regularly review and update your preparedness plans to ensure they remain relevant and effective. This proactive approach minimizes the stress associated with the unknown.

Break Down Larger Goals: Large-scale prepping goals can be overwhelming. Break them down into smaller, manageable tasks. Achieving these smaller tasks will provide a sense of accomplishment and help mitigate stress.

Family Communication: Maintain open communication with your family about your prepping efforts. Knowing that everyone is on the same page fosters a sense of unity and reduces the stress of potential misunderstandings during a crisis.

Connect with the Prepper Community: Join local or online prepper communities to share experiences and insights. Engaging with like-minded individuals provides a support system and a platform to discuss concerns, reducing the isolation that can contribute to stress.

Regular Training Drills: Familiarity breeds confidence. Regularly conduct training drills with your family to ensure everyone knows their roles and responsibilities. This familiarity reduces stress during actual emergencies.

Diversify Skills: Anxiety often stems from the fear of the unknown. Diversify your prepping skills to feel more capable and adaptable. Whether it's learning new cooking methods, gardening techniques, or self-defense strategies, acquiring diverse skills boosts confidence and reduces stress.

Celebrate Milestones: Acknowledge and celebrate prepping milestones. Whether it's reaching a specific stockpile quantity or successfully implementing a new security measure, celebrating achievements helps maintain a positive mindset and alleviate stress.

Create a Comfort Zone: Designate a space within your home as a prepping sanctuary. Having a well-organized and comforting space dedicated to your prepping activities can act as a stress-relief zone where you can focus on tasks without distractions.

Stay Informed, Not Overwhelmed: Stay informed about current events and potential threats, but avoid information overload. Limit exposure to stressful news and focus on actionable steps you can take to enhance your preparedness, reducing unnecessary anxiety.

Physical Exercise: Incorporate regular physical exercise into your routine. Physical activity is a proven stress-reliever, releasing endorphins that improve mood and reduce anxiety. Consider activities that align with prepping, such as hiking, gardening, or even home workout routines.

Build a Support Network: Share your prepping journey with friends and family who understand and support your efforts. Having a support network provides an outlet for discussing concerns and gaining valuable insights, reducing the emotional burden on an individual prepper.

Emergency Response Plan: Develop a clear emergency response plan and ensure that everyone in your family is familiar with it. Knowing you have a well-thought-out plan in place can alleviate stress by providing a structured approach to various scenarios.

Maintain a Positive Narrative: Frame your prepping efforts in a positive light. Instead of dwelling on potential doomsday scenarios, focus on the empowerment that comes from being self-sufficient and well-prepared. Shifting your mindset can significantly reduce stress.

Practice Relaxation Techniques: Learn and practice relaxation techniques such as progressive muscle relaxation, guided imagery, or aromatherapy. These techniques can help calm the mind and reduce stress levels, especially during high-pressure situations.

Financial Preparedness: Financial concerns can be a significant source of stress. Develop a budget and savings plan to ensure financial stability. Knowing you have financial resources set aside for emergencies provides a sense of security and reduces anxiety.

Regularly Evaluate Mental Well-being: Pay attention to your mental well-being. If stress and anxiety become overwhelming, don't hesitate to seek professional support. Mental health is a crucial aspect of overall preparedness, and addressing any issues early on can prevent them from escalating.

Connect with Nature: Spend time outdoors and connect with nature. Whether it's a walk in the woods, a camping trip, or tending to a garden, nature has a calming effect and can help alleviate stress associated with the hustle and bustle of daily life and prepping responsibilities.

Prepare for the Unexpected: Accept that uncertainties are inherent in life and preparedness efforts. Embrace the idea that not every scenario can be predicted or controlled.

Developing a mindset that is adaptable to change can reduce stress when faced with unexpected challenges.

By incorporating these stress and anxiety coping strategies into your prepping journey, you not only enhance your ability to navigate emergencies but also ensure that your mindset remains positive and focused on the well-being of your family during times of crisis. Remember, the journey of preparedness is as much about mental resilience as it is about physical readiness.

TRAINING DRILLS FOR FAMILY PREPAREDNESS

To minimize surprises during an emergency, regular family training drills are indispensable. Consider incorporating the following training drills into your prepper routine, and for this section I even included a tip:

Inventory Check Drill: Regularly assess and update your stockpile inventory. This ensures a comprehensive understanding of what is available and what requires replenishment.

Tip: Use this drill not only for inventory management, but also to educate your family on the importance of meticulous record-keeping and foresight in anticipating potential shortages. Lastly, this will allow for spoiled, outdated items to be revealed and ultimately replaced.

Emergency Cooking Challenge: Simulate scenarios where only pantry staples are available, utilizing alternative cooking methods like solar ovens or camp stoves.

Tip: This drill not only tests the adaptability of your family, but also familiarizes them with alternative cooking methods, ensuring they are comfortable and competent in using them when needed. It should get them familiar with the location of various items for cooking as well, especially if younger children are in your home. Alright, who's hungry?

Water Usage Simulation: Temporarily limit water usage to simulate scarcity, imparting the importance of conservation to your family.

Tip: Incorporate this drill into your routine to instill water conservation habits and educate your family on alternative water sources and purification methods. There is a good chance that a natural water source is near your home. Locate it now, so in an emergency you already have a plan to gather water from it to support your family.

Security Simulation: Conduct a home security drill to practice responses to potential threats, emphasizing communication and swift decision-making.

Tip: This drill goes beyond physical preparation and involves communication strategies. Analyze and refine your family's communication methods to enhance efficiency during emergencies.

BUILDING COMMUNITY AND SUPPORT NETWORKS

Establishing Trust with Like-minded Individuals

In the prepping realm, trust forms the bedrock of effective collaboration. When engaging with potential prepping allies, consider the following trust-building strategies:

Background Checks: Facilitate open discussions about prepping backgrounds and experiences, fostering an environment of transparency and trust.

Tip: Establish a framework for sharing information, ensuring that everyone feels comfortable disclosing essential details about their preparedness journey.

Skill Exchange: Organize skill-sharing activities such as workshops or classes, encouraging mutual learning and building trust through shared experiences.

Tip: Rotate the leadership of these workshops to showcase various skills within the community, fostering a sense of equality and shared responsibility.

Joint Drills: Collaborate on emergency drills to assess how well individuals and families work together. Practical experience is a powerful tool for evaluating trustworthiness.

Tip: During joint drills, observe not just the technical skills but also the interpersonal dynamics within groups, as effective collaboration during crises depends on both.

COMMUNITY EDUCATION OPPORTUNITIES

Investing in prepper education is a strategic move to fortify your community's preparedness. Local classes and workshops provide valuable opportunities for knowledge exchange. Consider the following educational avenues:

Budget Shopping Seminars: Gain insights into maximizing your budget when stockpiling essential items.

Tip: Leverage the expertise within your community to share innovative budgeting techniques and collectively identify cost-effective solutions.

Self-Defense Workshops: Equip community members with basic self-defense skills, ensuring safety during emergencies.

Tip: Encourage ongoing self-defense training, fostering a sense of empowerment within the community and reducing dependency on external security measures.

Gardening and Canning Classes: Explore sustainable practices like gardening and canning to supplement your pantry with fresh produce.

Tip: Collaborate with local experts to host advanced gardening workshops, delving into topics such as crop rotation, companion planting, and seed saving.

Firearm Safety Courses: Responsible gun ownership is integral to prepping. Engage in courses that teach proper firearm handling and safety.

Tip: Establish a community code of conduct regarding firearm safety, emphasizing responsible ownership and the importance of ongoing training.

In the intricate tapestry of prepper preparedness, the threads of a positive mindset and community collaboration weave a resilient fabric. By comprehending the psychology behind preparedness and fostering trust within your community, you fortify not only your pantry plan but also the collective strength of those around you. As we delve deeper into the heart of prepper survival, remember: the key to enduring any catastrophe lies not just in what you stockpile but in the strength of the minds and bonds that support it.

9

ADAPTING TO CHANGE: NAVIGATING SHIFTING SCENARIOS FOR 90-DAY SURVIVAL

"Waste not, want not."

— PROVERB

RESOURCEFULNESS AS A PREPPER

In the tapestry of the unforeseen, resourcefulness emerges as a beacon. Picture a prepper facing a temporary shortage of canned goods. Rather than succumbing to panic, they turn to pantry staples—rice, beans, and grains. Through culinary ingenuity, these staples transform into gourmet delights. In this final chapter, we unravel the art of adapting to change in our prepping journey.

Embrace Flexibility in Preparation Amidst Changing Conditions

Beyond our fortified 90-day nutritional survival food, envision a realm where unpredictability reigns—a prolonged power outage, disruptions in the supply chain, or unforeseen surges in demand for emergency supplies. Here, a prepper's ability to adapt becomes paramount.

SUPPLY CHAIN DISRUPTION

Scenario: Global events disrupt supply chains, limiting access to essential prepper pantry items.

Solution: In times of global disruptions affecting prepper pantry supplies, a key solution involves diversifying and expanding your stockpile. This means avoiding reliance on a single source, which boosts adaptability to unexpected challenges. Additionally, exploring local sourcing helps build community connections and reduces vulnerability to global supply chain issues. Another vital aspect is innovating alternative ways to secure essential items, ensuring a proactive response to scarcity. By adopting these measures, individuals can create a resilient and flexible preparedness strategy, navigating uncertainties with a more comprehensive approach.

Fostering strong connections within your local community forms the bedrock of a resilient prepper strategy, especially when it comes to securing essential supplies. To fortify your prepper pantry, consider establishing relationships with local farmers and producers. Building ties with these primary sources not only ensures a more direct and reliable supply chain, but also cultivates a sense of mutual support and cooperation. Investigating community-supported agriculture (CSA) programs further amplifies your self-sufficiency efforts. By participating in a CSA, you engage in a collaborative arrangement with local farmers, sharing in the risks and rewards of agricultural production. This not only bolsters your access to fresh and locally sourced produce, but also strengthens the community's overall food resilience. Additionally, embracing the practice of bartering with neighbors for needed supplies introduces a dynamic element of resource exchange. This not only promotes a spirit of communal assistance, but also diversifies the range of goods available within the community. Bartering becomes a symbiotic relationship where each prepper can contribute their unique skills or surplus items, fostering a network of interdependence that can be invaluable during times of scarcity. In essence, these interconnected relationships with local farmers, participation in CSA programs, and the practice of bartering with neighbors collectively weave a fabric of community resilience, ensuring that your prepper pantry is not only well-stocked but also intricately linked to the broader support network within your vicinity.

POWER OUTAGE PERSISTENCE

Scenario: An extended power outage challenges reliance on electronic tools for communication and sustenance.

Solution: In a situation where a prolonged power outage challenges our reliance on electronic tools, a key solution involves adding manual tools to our preparedness plan. This means incorporating items like hand-crank radios for communication and manual water pumps for a reliable water supply. Specific to the prepper pantry, keep the manual can opener and non-electric food processor! By diversifying our strategies in this way, we create a more robust and self-reliant approach to handling extended power disruptions, ensuring we can communicate and meet basic needs even when electronic tools are unavailable.

In the pursuit of comprehensive emergency preparedness, it is prudent to diversify your strategies for power sustainability. Investing in alternative power sources, such as solar chargers, emerges as a forward-thinking initiative to harness renewable energy. These devices not only contribute to a more sustainable and eco-friendly approach, but also offer a reliable means of charging essential electronic devices in the event of power outages. To bolster your preparedness even further, acquiring basic electrical repair skills proves invaluable. Equipping yourself with the knowledge to perform quick fixes empowers you to address minor electrical issues promptly, potentially restoring functionality to critical devices without undue delays. Additionally, implementing a rotating schedule for electronic device usage is a strategic measure to conserve energy and extend the operational life of your devices. This scheduling approach ensures that essential electronics are used judiciously, minimizing the strain on power sources and promoting long-term sustainability. By integrating these practices into your prepping regimen, you fortify your ability to navigate through unforeseen challenges with resilience and resourcefulness, ensuring that your power supply remains a reliable asset in times of crisis.

UNFORESEEN POPULATION SURGE

Scenario: An unexpected surge in individuals turning to prepping causes a demand upswing.

Solution: In a situation where more people are suddenly getting into prepping, and there's a rising demand for supplies, or a population boom, a key solution considers the broader context of increasing food demand. The United Nations predicts a 70% rise in food demand by 2050, making food storage and self-sufficiency crucial. The vital aspects of the solution involve regularly checking and adjusting your stockpile, tweaking quantities based on changing needs, and finding creative ways to ration resources for your family and community. One innovative approach is implementing a meal-sharing cooperative within your community. This involves collaborating with neighbors to rotate the responsibility of preparing meals for the group. By sharing resources and skills, each household contributes to the collective well-being, ensuring everyone has access to a variety of nutritious meals while minimizing individual strain on prepping supplies. Another creative rationing strategy involves establishing a community tool library. In a scenario where prepping supplies are in high demand, sharing tools and equipment can be more efficient than each household individually stockpiling them. Think *The Walking Dead* more like the Alexandria and Hilltop communities where tools were under lock and watch, but could be used by all. I'm sure some preppers are against this shared resource idea, barely trusting their neighbor right now for shovels. I get it, especially in an extended emergency situation, but it is in the "innovative approach" section as an idea. Remember, many hands make light work. This approach not only addresses the immediate surge in prepping interest but also prepares for the future challenges tied to the expected increase in global food demand.

To ensure the ongoing preparedness and sustainability of your prepper pantry, it is imperative to conduct regular stockpile audits. These assessments serve as a strategic measure to evaluate the status of your supplies, identify potential gaps, and adjust quantities accordingly. Simultaneously, implementing a community-wide rationing plan becomes a collaborative effort that not only fosters a sense of unity among prepper neighbors, but also ensures fair distribution of resources during prolonged emergencies. This collective approach enhances the resilience of the entire community, as each member contributes to and benefits from a shared pool of essential items. Furthermore, exploring cooperative gardening initiatives adds another layer of self-sufficiency. By joining forces with fellow preppers, you can create a communal space for cultivating crops, sharing responsibilities, and diversifying the types of produce available. This collaborative gardening effort not only contributes to the overall food security of the community, but also establishes a network of support, reinforcing the foundation of your prepping strategy. In the realm of rationing techniques for prolonged emergencies, these proactive measures underscore the significance of community collaboration and strategic planning, ensuring that your prepper pantry remains robust and resilient in the face of unforeseen challenges.

BASIC RATIONING TECHNIQUES

Basic food rationing techniques are vital for your prepper pantry stockpile. They help stretch your resources during uncertain times by controlling portions and prioritizing essentials. Rationing ensures your food lasts longer, providing sustained nourishment when faced with unexpected challenges.

Portion Control: Portion control stands as a cornerstone in the art of basic rationing. This technique involves meticulous planning and allocation of food items to optimize their usage over an extended period. Preppers can invest in measuring tools, such as kitchen scales and measuring cups, to precisely portion meals. By carefully managing portion sizes, prepper families can extend the lifespan of their stockpile, ensuring that every meal contributes to nutritional needs without unnecessary depletion of resources. Educating family members on the importance of portion control not only promotes efficiency, but also cultivates a mindful approach to consumption.

Meal Rotation: The strategy of meal rotation is a dynamic approach to basic rationing, ensuring a balanced and varied diet while maximizing the longevity of stored foods. Preppers can create a meal rotation schedule, systematically cycling through different recipes and ingredients. This not only prevents monotony in daily meals but also strategically uses versatile pantry staples. Experimenting with diverse and adaptable ingredients allows prepper families to explore various culinary possibilities, turning basic items into diverse and flavorful dishes. By implementing a thoughtful meal rotation plan, preppers can optimize nutrition and mitigate the risk of palate fatigue during prolonged emergencies.

These basic rationing techniques form the foundation of a prepper's food management strategy, emphasizing precision, variety, and adaptability. Through portion control and meal rotation, prepper families can navigate through extended survival scenarios with a strategic and sustainable approach to their stockpile, ensuring both physical well-being and mental resilience.

OUT-OF-THE-BOX RATIONING TECHNIQUES

In the intricate dance of prepping for unforeseen challenges, the art of rationing transcends the mundane, weaving together a tapestry of resilience and creativity within the prepper community. Here are a few unconventional rationing ideas you may have not considered:

Recipe Innovation: Embracing recipe innovation tran-scends the traditional boundaries of meal preparation during survival scenarios. This technique encourages preppers to view their pantry staples as versatile building blocks for creating diverse and nutritious meals. Hosting community recipe-sharing sessions becomes a collaborative effort where preppers exchange creative ideas to make the most out of limited resources. Compiling a recipe book for innovative meal ideas serves as a tangible resource, offering a catalog of inventive dishes crafted from basic pantry items. Through recipe innovation, preppers not only address nutritional needs but also inject a sense of culinary adventure into their emergency preparedness, transforming the act of rationing into a creative and community-building endeavor.

Community Collaboration: Out-of-the-box rationing extends beyond individual households, emphasizing the importance of community collaboration. Establishing a communal approach to rationing involves sharing resources and skills within the prepper community. Regular community meetings become platforms for discussing resource-sharing strategies, from ingredients to tools. Creating a skill-sharing database fosters a network where each prepper contributes unique skills, enhancing the collective ability to adapt and thrive. Through community collaboration, preppers not only fortify their own stockpiles but also create a resilient support system where the strengths of one complement the needs of another. This interconnected approach transforms the act of rationing from an individual challenge into a communal triumph, reinforcing the fabric of the prepper community.

As the prepper community navigates the complexities of rationing, these out-of-the-box techniques not only sustain nutritional needs but also cultivate a spirit of adaptability, turning the act of rationing into a communal victory against uncertainty.

CRAFTING RESILIENCE TO ENDURE AND THRIVE OVER THE LONG HAUL

Importance of Sound Mind, Sound Body

As the echoes of emergency scenarios linger, it is crucial to delve deeper into the symbiotic relationship between maintaining a sound mind and a healthy body throughout your prepper journey. Exercise transforms into more than just a physical fitness routine; it emerges as the cornerstone for fostering mental acuity and fortitude. Engaging in daily walks, cultivating a garden, or performing regular home maintenance exercises not only contribute to the well-being of your body, but also serve as powerful tools for sharpening the mind. These activities become indispensable components, enhancing the efficiency and effectiveness of your prepper activities.

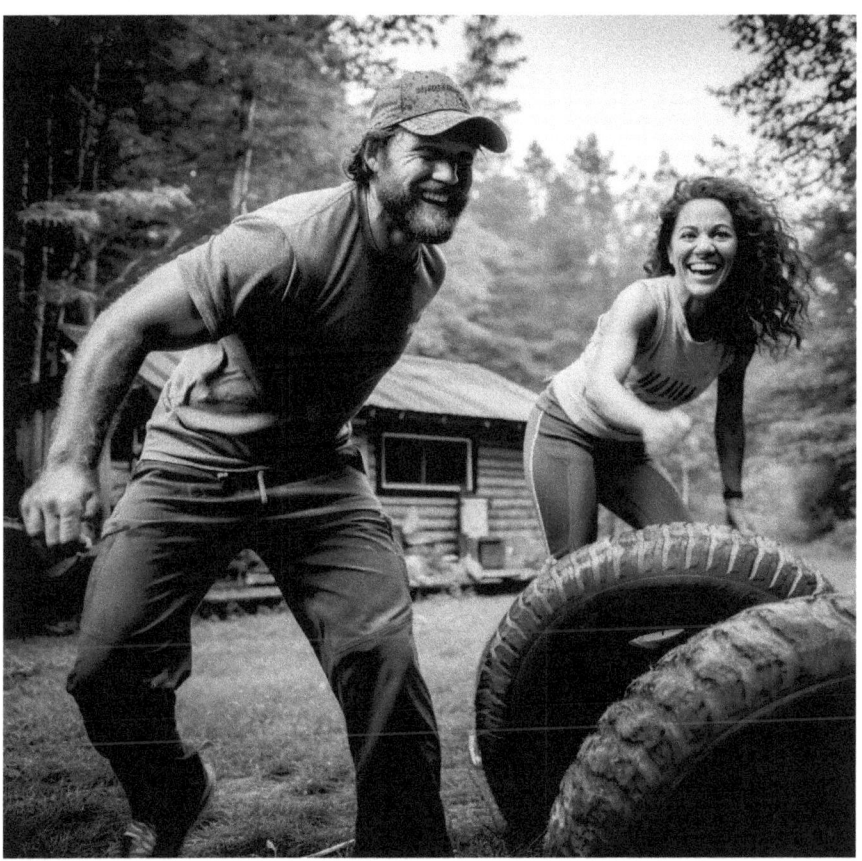

ELABORATING ON PHYSICAL FITNESS

Daily Walks: Incorporate daily walks not only as a cardio-vascular exercise but as an opportunity for mental rejuvenation.

Explore different routes to add variety and stimulate your senses.

Use this time for reflective thinking and mental preparedness.

Gardening: Cultivate a garden not only for food production but as a therapeutic space for physical activity. Experiment with diverse crops to nurture a sense of curiosity and adaptability.

Engage family members in gardening, fostering a shared connection with the earth.

Home Maintenance: View home maintenance tasks as more than chores; consider them as functional workouts. Rotate tasks to target different muscle groups, promoting overall physical fitness. Use maintenance time as an opportunity to assess and enhance the security of your living space.

THE SPIRIT OF LIFELONG PREPAREDNESS

The prepper ethos goes beyond the immediate concerns of physical preparedness. It transcends into the spirit of lifelong learning, marking a commitment to continuous personal development. Establishing a home library becomes not just a storage of books but a sanctuary of knowledge covering a diverse range of subjects. From classic literature and instructional guides, to cutting-edge educational resources, your library becomes a dynamic source of empowerment and enrichment.

Lifelong Learning

Home Library: Build a comprehensive home library, curating books that span various subjects.

Include classic literature for cultural enrichment and a deeper understanding of human nature.

Incorporate instructional guides and educational resources to hone practical skills.

E-books and Audiobooks: Explore the world of ebooks and audiobooks for a modern and diverse learning experience. Utilize digital resources to access a wide array of topics and perspectives.

Foster a culture of shared reading within your prepper community.

Natural Medicine: Delve deeper into the basics of natural medicine and herbal remedies.

Cultivate a medicinal herb garden as a hands-on learning experience.

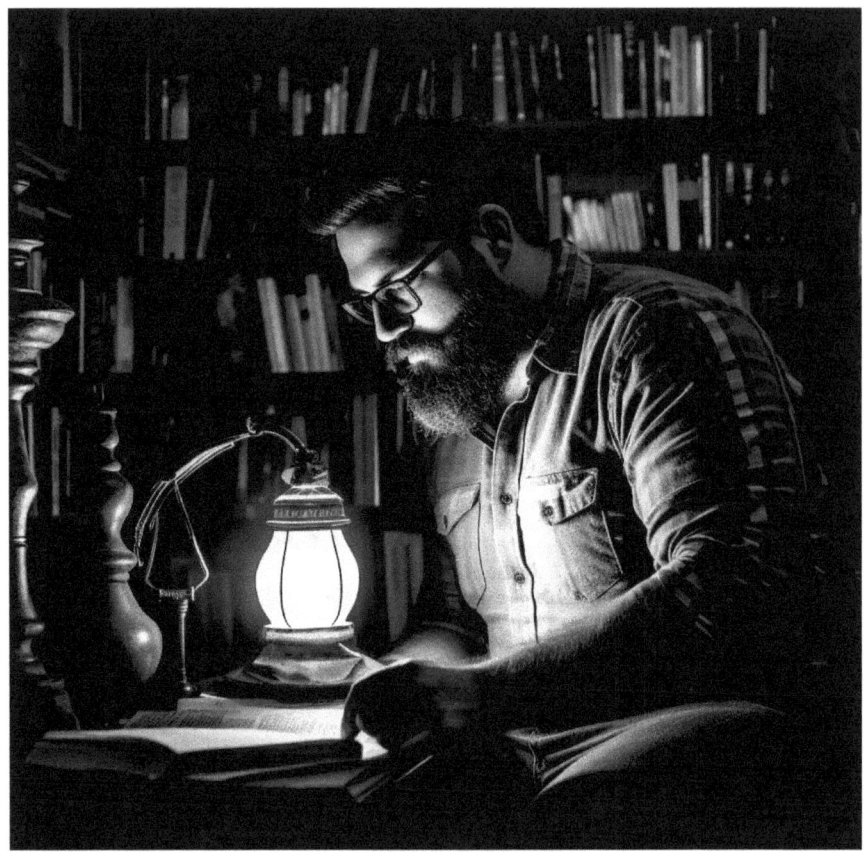

Attend workshops or online courses focused on herbal medicine to broaden your expertise.

First Aid Training: Enhance your first aid skills through advanced training programs.

Enroll in certified first aid courses with a specific focus on emergency scenarios.

Invest in high-quality first aid supplies and regularly practice using them for proficiency.

A Few More for the Road: Flexibility is the heartbeat of the prepper lifestyle. Consider alternative communication methods, such as a HAM radio, as traditional lines may falter during crises. Embrace a manual water pump to overcome potential power shortages. Rotate your garden harvest strategically, adapting to fluctuating supply chains. These adjustments aren't hurdles but milestones. As you've journeyed toward self-sustainability, these adaptive measures are your future strengths to lifelong learning.

THE UNSEEN STRENGTH IN ADAPTABILITY

As we conclude this prepper odyssey, reflect on the profound truth that adaptation is not a mere concession, but a powerful demonstration of strength. Life's surprises, when met with a flexible mindset, cease to be burdens; they transform into opportunities for growth and resilience. Armed with knowledge, resourcefulness, and a resilient spirit, the prepper isn't merely surviving in the face of uncertainty; they are thriving. Adapting to change isn't a burden in the ultimate prepper's journey—it's the unwritten chapter where unforeseen challenges become stepping stones toward enduring survival. Embrace the surprises life brings, for they are often better than the things we think we see coming!

A FINAL WORD

Your Path to Resilience

As we draw the final curtain on this journey, it's not the end but a new beginning. Through the chapters of "The Ultimate Prepper Pantry Survival Guide," you've ventured into a world of preparedness, transforming fear into strength and vulnerability into empowerment. You've embraced the art of stockpiling, ensuring your family's well-being even in the face of the most daunting of circumstances. You've made the pledge to never again be caught unprepared, to shield your loved ones from the unpredictable and thrive in adversity.

You've discovered that true preparedness is not about fear; it's about empowerment. It's about seizing control of your future, shattering the shackles of uncertainty, and awakening your inner reservoir of resilience. It is the profound under-standing that you are the architect of your family's safety, the guardian of their well-being, and the weaver of a future adorned with the vibrant threads of hope and security.

Throughout this journey, you've learned that building a prepper pantry is not merely an act of stockpiling—it's an act of love. It's a promise to your family, a commitment to their protection, and a demonstration of your unwavering dedication. You've understood that preparedness is not a chore but a calling, a calling to safeguard the lives you hold most dear.

But why did you choose to follow me on this transformational path? Well my authority in preparedness is not solely based on expertise, but also on my profound empathy for the fears and anxieties unpreparedness can inflict. With an understanding of your concerns, I have guided you through this journey, offering practical advice and unwavering support.

When you contemplate the wealth of knowledge you've amassed, remember that preparedness is not merely a goal—it is a way of life. It's a vow that you will always be ready, a pledge that your family will always be secure, and the embodiment of resilience. It is the promise of a future where you approach each day with confidence, knowing you have mastered the art of preparedness. Your family is no longer exposed to the whims of fate; they are sheltered within the fortress of your prepper pantry.

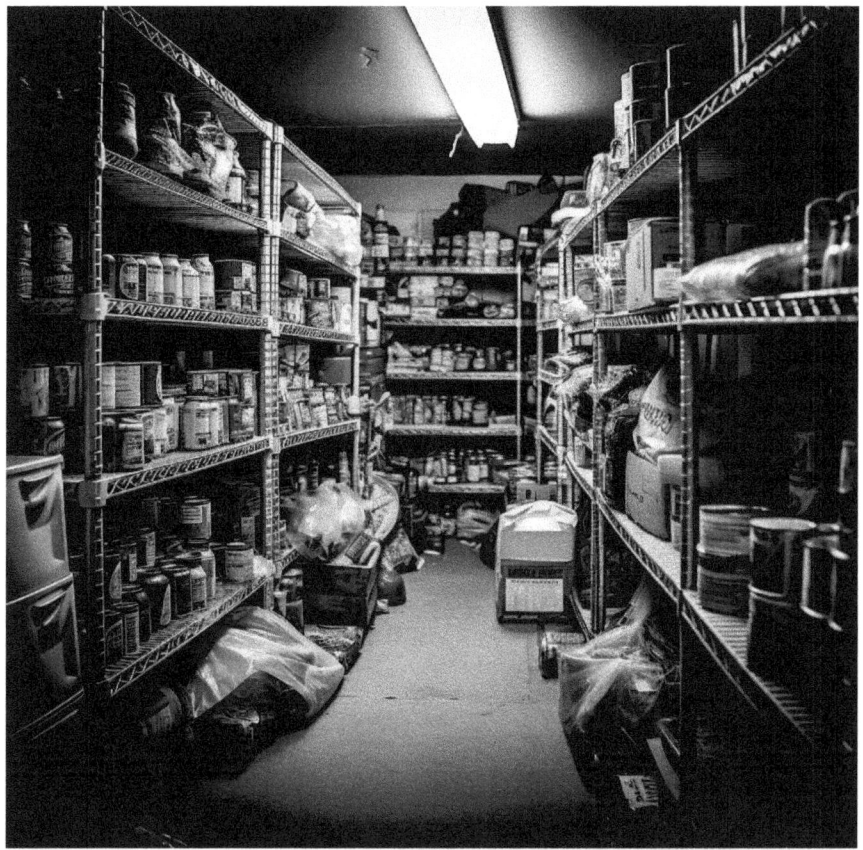

So, as you close this book, do not say farewell to the principles it imparts; instead, carry them with you as you step into a brighter, safer future. Your path to resilience is not a solitary one; it's a legacy that will be passed on to your loved ones. May you, your family, and generations to come find solace in the knowledge that, together, you are prepared for anything and capable of thriving amidst any challenge.

Embrace your journey, be the guardian of your family's safety, and stand as a beacon of hope in a world that may yet be uncertain. Your destiny of preparedness awaits, and with me as your guide, your future is bright, secure, and filled with the vibrant hues of preparedness and peace of mind. Stay prepared friends!

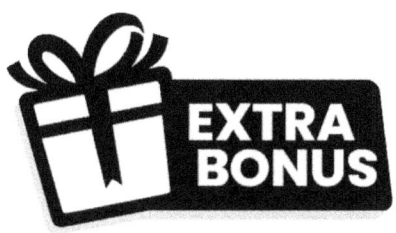

Thank you for embarking on this literary journey with me! Your support and enthusiasm for my book mean the world. As a token of gratitude, I'm thrilled to offer you exclusive access to the "Ultimate Prepper Pantry Inventory Calculator Spreadsheet." Simply scan the QR code below and drop your email to receive this invaluable tool – no strings attached, just a little something extra for being a loyal reader. Your continued support is truly appreciated, and I hope this bonus enriches your prepping journey in the most extraordinary ways!

▽ SCAN THE QR CODE BELOW ▽

SCAN ME

SCAN THE QR CODE BELOW

As an independent author with a small marketing budget, reviews are my livelihood on this platform. I would be incredibly thankful if you could take just 60 seconds to write a brief review on Amazon, even if it's just a few sentences!

You can do so by scanning the QR code taking you to my author page on Amazon. Find this book to review, or shop for other best-sellers in my prepping collection! I do love hearing from my readers, and I personally read every single review. Thank you for the support!

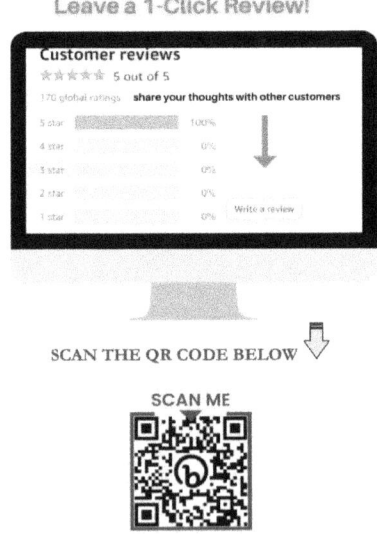

REFERENCES

The Ultimate Prepper Pantry Survival Guide

CHAPTER 1:https://www.emergencyprepgear.com/food-storage-and-production

https://theprepared.com/homestead/guides/supermarket-food-list/

https://www.samhsa.gov/find-help/disaster-distress-helpline/disaster-types

https://theprovidentprepper.org/raising-confident-self-reliant-kid-preppers-14-essential-skills/

https://theprovidentprepper.org/food-storage-for-the-healthy-minded/

CHAPTER   2:https://thehomesteadinghippy.com/survival-stockpile/

https://ezprepping.com/how-many-calories-you-need-to-survive-free-calculator/

https://extension.oregonstate.edu/catalog/pub/em-9331-survival-basics-food

https://theprovidentprepper.org/top-10-foods-to-hoard-for-the-end-of-the-world-as-we-know-it/

https://themakinglife.com/food-preservation-methods/

https://acrelife.com/must-have-food-preservation-tools-and-equipment

https://homesteadingfamily.com/building-up-your-long-term-food-storage-supply/

https://www.new-terra-natural-food.com/cheap-survival-food.html

https://www.tactical.com/survival-food-storage-basics/

https://theprovidentprepper.org/how-to-package-dry-foods-in-mylar-bags-for-long-term-storage/

https://theprovidentprepper.org/packaging-dry-foods-in-glass-jars-for-long-term-food-storage/

https://theprovidentprepper.org/packaging-dry-foods-in-plastic-bottles-for-long-term-food-storage/

https://www.survivopedia.com/small-spaces-stockpile/

https://www.happypreppers.com/water.html

https://survivalistprepper.net/25-multi-use-prepping-supplies-survival-tools/

https://theprovidentprepper.org/30-day-grid-down-cooking-challenge-lessons-learned-and-fuel-usage/

https://prepared-housewives.com/extreme-menu-planning/

https://docs.google.com/spreadsheets/d/1VNmScOMok784FVKdFBSQ70O-N7G1kGVXIDRYKRtb16w/edit?usp=drive_link

https://prepared-housewives.com/extreme-menu-planning/

https://www.youtube.com/watch?v=kKIfgsCH4Kc

https://theprepared.com/prepping-basics/guides/fifo/

https://thehomesteadinghippy.com/ways-to-tell-food-is-spoiled/

https://www.foodstoragemoms.com/what-to-do-with-your-old-stockpile-of-food/

https://theprovidentprepper.org/best-strategies-for-growing-a-reliable-survival-garden/

https://theprovidentprepper.org/how-to-store-seeds-to-achieve-the-highest-germination-rate-and-plant-vigor/

https://www.offthegridnews.com/extreme-survival/the-absolute-best-protein-sources-when-society-ends-as-we-know-it/

https://www.primalsurvivor.net/wilderness-survival-food/

https://theprovidentprepper.org/community-a-critical-link-to-survival/

https://www.survivalsullivan.com/hide-your-preps/

https://thesurvivalmom.com/creative-storage-solutions-stash/

https://www.quora.com/What-laws-would-you-observe-during-The-Apocalypse

https://survivalistprepper.net/home-defense-tactics-home-security/

https://theprovidentprepper.org/a-preppers-guide-to-communicating-in-an-emergency/#:~:text=During%20an%20emergency%2C%20you%20may,old%20fashioned%20hand%2Dwritten%20notes.

https://valor.militarytimes.com/hero/8193

https://www.happypreppers.com/survival-psychology.html

https://prepperspriority.com/psychological-resilience-for-preppers-and-survivalists/

https://thesurvivalmom.com/try-it-today-preparedness-drills-kids/

https://prepared-housewives.com/6-subjects-preppers-should-learn/

https://www.foodstoragemoms.com/how-to-be-tougher-mentally-as-a-prepper/#:~:text=Physical%20fitness%20goes%20hand%20in,be%20a%20strong%2Dminded%20prepper!

https://theprovidentprepper.org/long-term-food-storage-creative-solutions-to-build-a-critical-asset/

https://www.theorganicprepper.com/survival-of-the-most-adapatable/

https://thesurvivalsummit.com/establishing-a-comprehensive-p-a-c-e-plan-for-survival-preparedness/

Lighthouse Survival on Facebook:

https://www.facebook.com/profile.php?id=100087989030621

www.ingramcontent.com/pod-product-compliance
Lightning Source LLC
Chambersburg PA
CBHW051617120626
46551CB00014B/1838